THE MIRACLE GASTRITIS COOKBOOK: 150+ Easy, Delicious, and Gastritis-Friendly Recipes to Cure Gastritis, Heal Your Stomach, and Prevent Gastritis

Lydia G. Perez

All rights reserved. No part of this publication may be reproduced, distributed, or transmitted in any form or by any means, including photocopying, recording, or other electronic or mechanical methods, without the prior written permission of the publisher, except in the case of brief quotations embodied in critical reviews and certain other noncommercial uses permitted by copyright law. Copyright © Lydia G. Perez, 2023.

TABLE OF CONTENTS

INTRODUCTION

CHAPTER ONE

CHAPTER TWO

CHAPTER THREE

CHAPTER FOUR

CHAPTER FIVE

CHAPTER SIX

CHAPTER SEVEN

CHAPTER EIGHT

CHAPTER NINE

CHAPTER TEN

CHAPTER ELEVEN

EPILOGUE

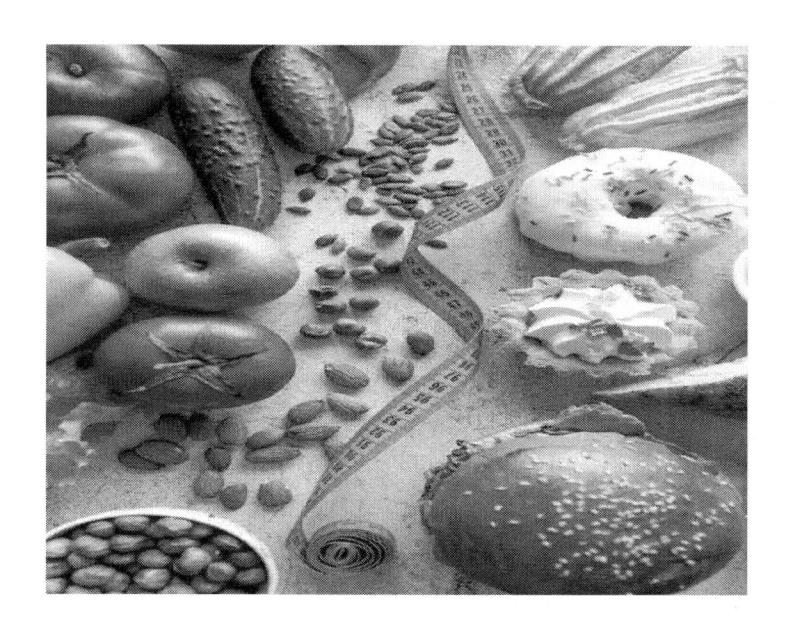

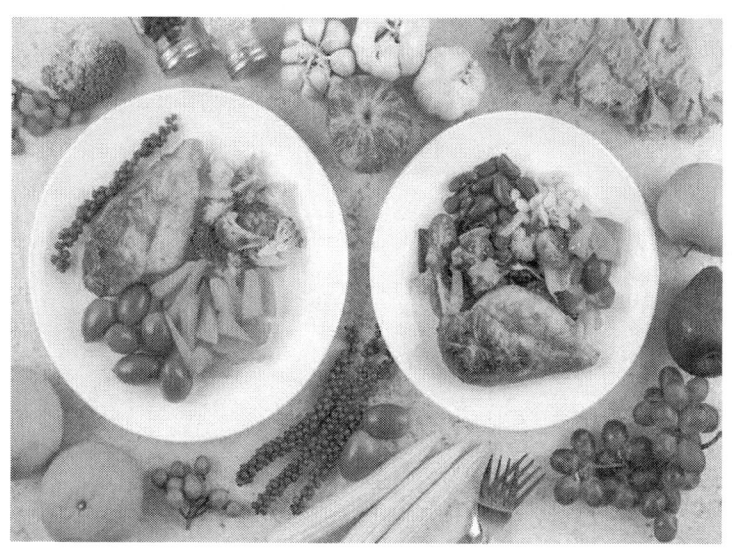

INTRODUCTION

Introduction to Gastritis and Diet Management

Just try to picture a life without illness or other health issues, where you don't even need medical attention. You must be asking yourself, "How is this even possible?" But it is, and all you need to do is alter your way of life to make it healthier. But although it's true that junk food is enticing and tough to resist, what about the gas or acidity that you experience later on when you switch to a gastritis diet?

Thus, it is never too late to begin anything or to begin making progress toward your goal of leading a healthy life. Let's get going. People often have problems with gastritis. It is an irritation, erosion, or inflammation of the stomach's lining. However, it begins as an acute disease that has the potential to become chronic. Or, to put it another way, gastritis occurs when the stomach's lining becomes disrupted, which then triggers the release of acids. causes of gastric problems.

However, there may be a number of causes for gastrointestinal problems. Below are a few who are often at fault.

1. Upper Intestinal Gas: Aerophagia is the practice of swallowing gas, which may take the following forms: snorting gum loose dentures Smoking straws while drinking or eating too quickly

2. Lower Intestinal Gas: This occurs when intestinal bacteria react with the large intestine's undigested food, causing gas to be expelled from the body in the form of flatulence.

These foods consist of foods high in starch, such as maize, potatoes, and pasta. spicy and fatty dishes Cabbage, beans, onions, and asparagus are among the vegetables. fruit such as peaches, pears, and apples, having an extended period of an empty stomach, indulging in excessively hot meals, or abusing alcohol.

One of the main causes of this issue is taking on too much stress, tension, and worry. Another key cause is a disruption in mental health. Additionally, you run the risk of developing a gas issue if you don't chew your meal well. Helicobacter pylori (H. pylori) is a bacterium that lives in the mucous lining of the stomach and, if left untreated, may result in stomach cancer or ulcers.

Another cause of gastritis is bile reflux, in which bile from the biliary duct backflows into the stomach. Acidity, indigestion, bloating, heartburn, bacterial infection, constipation, and other factors are additional explanations that you should not disregard. Gastritis Problems and Symptoms.

The most typical symptoms of having gas in the stomach are listed for you. There may be other symptoms as well, but these are the most frequent ones.

Treatment and Diagnosis of Gastric Issues

There are certain tests that must be performed to determine the source of any health issue, and difficulties with gastritis are no exception. Upright endoscopy. This procedure, also known as an esophagogastroduodenoscopy or OGD, involves the examination of your stomach, small intestine, and esophagus. The doctor inserts an endoscope, a small, flexible tube, into your mouth. It travels down your neck and into your stomach, intestines, and food pipe.

Additionally, a camera is attached to the tube's end, allowing for a full view of the stomach and intestines. a blood test Doctors do blood tests in order to identify causes, symptoms, and other conditions. The bacteria Helicobacter pylori (H. pylori), which is often the cause of gastrointestinal issues, may be recommended by physicians. Fecal Occult Blood Test or Stool

Test A stool culture determines if any bacteria that might exacerbate gastritis symptoms are present in the digestive system.

However, therapy begins after the cause and stage have been identified. How to Treat Gastritis Medication and dietary adjustments are part of the treatment. Poor diet food is beneficial for stomach-related issues. A bland diet for gastritis is what? It is a short-term eating regimen made up of simple-to-digest meals that are easy on the stomach and digestive system. However, is a diet program helpful for gastritis? Yes, as we will describe in the next part, a well-designed food plan is quite helpful for controlling and lowering the symptoms of gastritis.

Along with dietary adjustments, your doctor may suggest certain drugs. To lessen stomach acid, doctors may prescribe antacids and other medications. You will be given drugs to treat heartburn if the gastritis was brought on by a viral or bacterial illness.

Inflammation of the stomach lining is a characteristic of the frequent digestive ailment known as gastritis. It may result in a variety of symptoms with varying degrees of severity and persistence. It is essential to comprehend these signs in order to diagnose gastritis early and treat it effectively. In this post, we shall examine the main signs and symptoms of gastritis.

1. Abdominal pain: Abdominal discomfort or pain is one of the defining signs of gastritis. This discomfort in the upper abdomen might vary from a subtle aching to a severe, scorching feeling. It often feels like a gnawing or cramping sensation, and certain meals may make it worse.

2. Vomiting and Nausea Constant nausea and, in some circumstances, vomiting are side effects of gastroenteritis. Whether it happens just after eating or on an empty stomach, nausea may range from moderate to severe. More often than not, people with severe gastritis may vomit.

3. Gas and bloating: Bloating and increased gas production are common symptoms of gastroenteritis. This could make you feel uncomfortable and full. Abdominal discomfort may be exacerbated by bloating, which tends to get worse after meals.

4. Lack of appetite: Gastritis may cause a decrease in appetite, making it difficult to eat regular meals. The pain and nausea brought on by the disease may cause a loss of appetite.

5. Indigestion: Gastritis often manifests as heartburn, which is characterized by a burning feeling in the chest or neck. It could happen if the esophagus is irritated by stomach acid. Heartburn may be a sign of gastritis, but it is more often related to gastroesophageal reflux disease (GERD).

6. Digestive System: Dyspepsia, another name for indigestion, is a broad word for pain or discomfort in the upper abdomen. It may include a variety of signs and symptoms, including

bloating, fullness, and burning. Patients with gastritis often complain of indigestion.

7. Bloody or dark stools: Gastritis sometimes causes bleeding in the stomach lining, which may cause black or tarry stools. In more serious cases, the bleeding may be more considerable, resulting in bright red or bloody stools or vomit.

8. Tiredness: The absorption of certain minerals, notably iron and vitamin B12, might be hampered by chronic gastritis. As a consequence of vitamin shortages, people with gastritis may feel weak or even have anemia.

9. Losing Weight: People with severe or persistent gastritis may unintentionally lose weight. A drop in body weight may result from the interaction of decreased appetite, sickness, and poor food absorption.

10. Chest discomfort While gastritis predominantly affects the stomach, it may sometimes result in discomfort or pain in the

chest. Chest discomfort should always be evaluated by a doctor since it might be mistaken for heart-related problems.

It's crucial to remember that each individual will experience gastritis symptoms differently. While some people may just feel a little pain, others can have more severe and enduring effects. Furthermore, whereas the symptoms of chronic gastritis might appear gradually over time, those of acute gastritis can appear suddenly and intensely.

If you think you may have gastritis or are exhibiting any of these symptoms, it is best to see a doctor for a correct diagnosis, advice on treatment, and recommendations for dietary changes. Understanding the underlying reason is essential for efficient therapy of gastroenteritis since it may be brought on by a variety of things, such as an infection, certain drugs, alcohol intake, and stress.

Avoiding certain foods may assist with gastritis symptoms and encourage the repair of the stomach lining. These foods should be avoided if you have gastritis:

1. Spicy foods include: Spices and hot spices may aggravate the symptoms of gastritis by irritating the stomach lining. Steer clear of foods that include a lot of black pepper, spicy sauce, or chili peppers.

2. Foods with Acidity: Acidic meals and drinks may cause the stomach to produce more acid, making gastritis worse. Citrus fruits (such oranges and lemons), tomatoes, and tomato-based goods like spaghetti sauce are among examples.

3. Fatty and fried foods: High-fat and fried meals are more difficult to digest and may cause pain by delaying the emptying of the stomach. Avoid fried foods like chicken, fries, and greasy fast food.

4. Carbonated Beverages: Carbonated beverages, such as soda and sparkling water, may exacerbate the symptoms of gastritis by causing bloating and gas.

5. Caffeine: Caffeinated beverages including coffee, tea, and sodas might accelerate the formation of stomach acid, which could exacerbate the symptoms of gastritis. If you prefer decaffeinated versions of these drinks, choose them.

6. Alcohol: Alcohol may aggravate gastritis symptoms by irritating the stomach lining. Do not consume alcoholic drinks such as beer, wine, or liquor.

7. Processed and Spicy Meats: Sausage and pepperoni are two examples of processed meats that often have high fat content and seasonings that might aggravate gastritis symptoms.

8. Foods with Lots of Seasoning: For those with gastritis, foods that rely heavily on spices, garlic,

and onions might be troublesome. These spices may be unpleasant to the stomach.

9. Milk and Dairy Products: Due to lactose intolerance, some people with gastritis may have difficulty digesting dairy products. Acid production may also be induced by dairy. Think about lactose-free or non-dairy substitutes.

10. Chocolate: Chocolate doubles as a gastritis trigger since it includes both fat and caffeine. Steer clear of chocolate bars and anything containing cocoa.

11. Peppermint and mint: The lower esophageal sphincter may be loosened by mint and peppermint, which can worsen symptoms by allowing stomach acid to flow back into the esophagus. This includes mint-flavored candy and peppermint tea.

12. Foods that are processed and high in sugar Sugary snacks, sweets, and highly processed meals may raise blood sugar levels and make

you feel uncomfortable. Limit sugary snacks and choose healthy, unadulterated meals instead.

13. Big Meals: Overeating may strain the stomach even more and make the symptoms of gastritis worse. In the course of the day, choose to eat smaller, more frequent meals.

14. Raw vegetables: Although veggies are typically good for you, raw ones may be difficult to digest and may cause stomach discomfort. Vegetables may be more palatable by being steamed or cooked.

15. Foods that are canned or pickled: Foods in cans and pickles often have high salt content and preservative levels, which can irritate the lining of the stomach.

Keep in mind that everyone has a different level of tolerance, so what causes symptoms in one person may not have the same effect on another. It's crucial to maintain a food journal to track particular triggers, and you should speak with a healthcare provider for individualized dietary advice depending on the severity and underlying reasons of your gastritis.

Managing gastritis and fostering stomach healing both need dietary changes. Overview of Gastritis Inflammation of the stomach lining is the defining characteristic of the common gastrointestinal illness known as gastritis. Since it contains the glands that secrete stomach acid and the digestive enzymes required to break down food, this apparently harmless lining is crucial to the digestive process.

If this lining becomes inflamed, it may cause a variety of unpleasant symptoms and, if untreated, may result in more serious consequences. Gastritis may present itself in a variety of ways, from acute and transient to chronic and persistent. Those who may be impacted by this disorder or who want to stop it from happening must be aware of its causes, symptoms, and possible effects.

Here, we dig into a thorough overview of gastritis. causes and precipitants Although there are many different causes of gastritis, they may be generally divided into the following significant factors:

1. Infection with Helicobacter pylori (H. pylori): The presence of H. pylori, a bacteria that may infiltrate the stomach lining and produce inflammation, is one of the most frequent causes of gastritis. Antibiotic therapy is often necessary to eradicate this illness.

2. NSAIDs (non-steroidal anti-inflammatory drugs) Regular use of NSAIDs, such as aspirin and ibuprofen, may cause gastritis by irritating the stomach lining. Careful monitoring is necessary while using these drugs on a regular basis.

3. Excessive Alcohol Consumption Alcohol may irritate and damage the stomach lining, which can aggravate gastritis.

4. Autoimmune responses: Autoimmune gastritis may occur when the body's immune system accidentally attacks the stomach lining. This illness may affect the stomach's capacity to manufacture necessary compounds like intrinsic factor, which is necessary for absorbing vitamin B12.

5. Stress: Chronic stress may increase the symptoms of gastritis, even if it is not a direct cause.

6. Gastroenteritis Symptoms: Numerous symptoms of gastritis often appear, and each person will experience these symptoms differently in terms of intensity and length.

Typical signs include:
Abdominal Pain: Gastritis is characterized by a chronic, dull pain or burning feeling in the upper abdomen. This ache could become worse after eating or while you're starving. Vomiting and Nausea Gastritis may cause nausea and, in rare circumstances, vomiting.

Gas and bloating: Many people with gastritis have more bloating and gas than usual, which causes them to feel full and uncomfortable.

Loss of appetite: Because of the pain and nausea it might cause, gastroenteritis can reduce appetite.

Heartburn Heartburn, which is characterized by a burning feeling in the chest or neck, may occur in some people with gastritis.

Diagestion: Dyspepsia, or indigestion, is a frequent problem that may include a number of symptoms, such as bloating, a feeling of fullness, and pain. Bloody or dark stools: When gastritis is severe, the stomach lining might bleed, which can cause black or tarry stools.

Fatigue and Loss of Weight: Chronic gastritis may make it difficult for nutrients to be absorbed, which might result in vitamin deficits that cause weakness, exhaustion, or weight loss.

Treatment and administration: Gastritis is often treated by treating the underlying cause, providing symptom relief, and avoiding recurrence.

Among the possible treatment plans are:

Medications Proton pump inhibitors (PPIs), antibiotics (for H. pylori), or antacids may be recommended, depending on the underlying reason.

Dietary Modifications: Adopting a gastritis-friendly diet may help control symptoms and encourage recovery by avoiding irritants like hot and acidic foods. Stress management Including stress-reduction strategies like mindfulness or relaxation exercises might be helpful.

Avoiding Triggers: It's essential to recognize and stay away from triggers like alcohol and NSAIDs to stop gastritis flare-ups.

Monitoring and Follow-Up: To measure progress and modify treatment regimens as necessary, regular medical checkups and monitoring of gastritis symptoms are crucial.

In conclusion, gastritis is a digestive disorder that, if left untreated, may have a substantial negative influence on a person's quality of life. Understanding its origins, identifying its symptoms, and getting help as soon as possible from a doctor are essential for treating gastritis efficiently and avoiding problems. People with gastritis may effectively manage the condition and enjoy better digestive health by adopting lifestyle modifications, following medication regimens, and making educated food decisions.

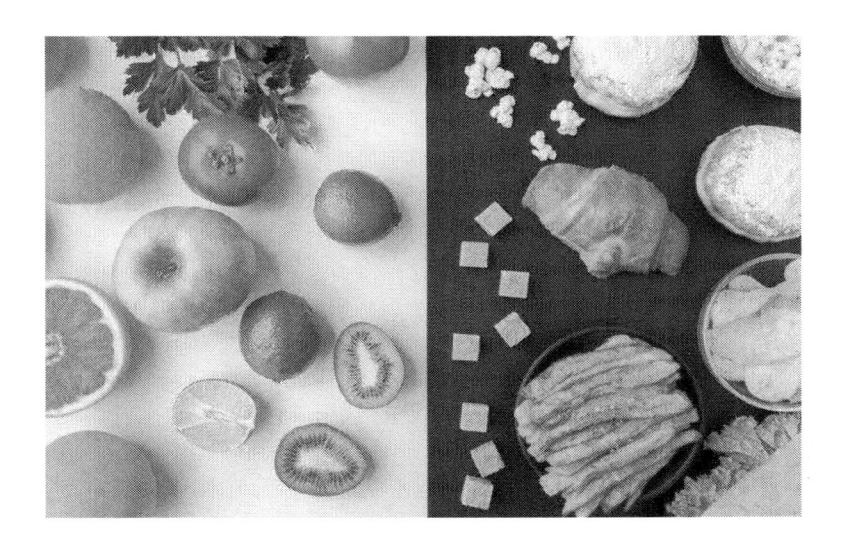

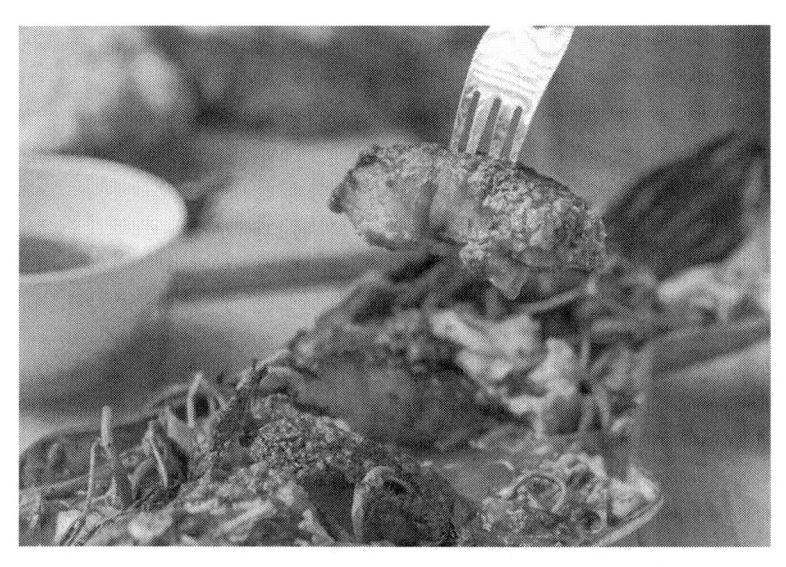

CHAPTER ONE

Gastritis-Friendly Foods and Ingredients

Getting Started with Gastritis-Friendly Foods Gastritis, a disorder characterized by stomach lining irritation, may cause pain and disturbances in everyday life. However, one of your most effective management strategies for gastritis is right at your fingertips: the foods you choose to eat.

The first step to easing symptoms and promoting stomach health is to comprehend the fundamentals of meals that are good for people with gastritis. A person with gastritis may have different dietary requirements depending on the severity and underlying reasons of their ailment, but there are general principles that may guide food choices for better health.

Foods that are good for people with gastroparesis are often ones that are easy on the stomach and reduce inflammation rather than exacerbate it. These meals are designed to provide necessary nutrients, encourage healing, and lessen discomfort.

Here are some essential guidelines to keep in mind:

1. Low-Acidity Options: High-acid foods may aggravate the stomach lining, which is already delicate, increasing pain and symptoms. Low-acid meals that are suitable for people with gastroenteritis often include non-citrus fruits (such as apples and bananas), non-tomato vegetables (such as spinach and carrots), and non-citrus fruit juices (such as apple juice).

2. Anti-Inflammatory Treatments: Anti-inflammatory foods may be consumed to reduce gastritis-related inflammation. These meals often include fatty fish like salmon and mackerel that are high in omega-3 fatty acids, nutritious grains like oats and brown rice, and different herbs and spices with

anti-inflammatory effects like ginger and turmeric.

3. Foods High in Fiber for Gastritis: A diet that is good for those with gastritis should include dietary fiber. It encourages normal digestion and may aid in preventing constipation, which is a typical problem for people with gastritis. You may incorporate high-fiber meals like whole grains, oats, and soluble fiber sources like apples and bananas.

4. Lean protein choices include: Although choosing the right protein sources is important for treating gastritis, protein is also necessary for good health in general. Choose lean proteins such as skinless chicken, lean beef, tofu, and lentils. These choices are less likely to cause pain and are easy on the stomach.

5. Light and non-spicy foods: Mild tastes are a common characteristic of meals that are good for people with gastroenteritis. Use spices and other hot components sparingly, if at all. Instead,

concentrate on utilizing mild spices like fresh herbs, lemon zest, and a dash of olive oil to improve the flavor of your food without upsetting your palate.

6. Gentle beverages for gastritis: For digestive health, staying hydrated is essential, but not all liquids are healthy for those with gastritis. Avoid alcohol, fizzy drinks, and caffeine-containing beverages since they may make your symptoms worse. Choose non-citrus fruit juices, water, and herbal teas like chamomile and peppermint instead.

An essential part of controlling this ailment is comprehending the principles of meals that are favorable to people with gastritis. You may lessen the chance that your gastritis symptoms will worsen and encourage the repair of your stomach lining by choosing meals that follow these guidelines. To develop a customized gastritis-friendly diet plan catered to your unique requirements and tastes, it is advised to speak with a healthcare provider or a qualified dietitian.

However, it is crucial to realize that individual tolerances may differ. You can actively work towards better gut health and enhanced wellbeing by making the proper dietary choices. A person with gastritis may have different dietary requirements depending on the severity and underlying reasons of their ailment, but there are general principles that may help direct food choices for better health.

Fruits:

Apples: Apples stand out as a particularly good option for those with gastritis because of their low acidity. Without putting too much strain on the stomach, they provide fiber and natural sweetness.

Bananas: Bananas are a fantastic choice for a snack or addition to breakfast because they are high in potassium and simple to digest.

Pears: Pears are less acidic than many other fruits and have a mild, sweet flavor. They provide a good amount of dietary fiber as well.

Melons: Low-acid fruits like watermelon, cantaloupe, and honeydew can hydrate you while being easy on your stomach.

Vegetables:

Rotaries: A versatile and low-acid vegetable option is carrots. They are a fantastic source of beta-carotene and can be eaten raw or cooked.

Spinach: Leafy green spinach is typically well tolerated by people with gastritis. It contains a lot of minerals and vitamins. Zucchini said: A mild and non-acidic vegetable, zucchini can be used as a substitute for pasta or in a variety of other dishes.

Grains:

Oats: When made into oatmeal, oats are a whole grain that offers dietary fiber and can be a calming option for the stomach.

Brown Rice: The base of many meals that are suitable for people with gastritis can be made with brown rice, a low-acid substitute for white rice.

Dairy and dairy substitutes:

Almond Milk: Almond milk is a non-dairy substitute that can be used in place of regular milk and is typically low in acidity.

Yogurt: Even though some people with gastritis may have issues with dairy, plain yogurt with live cultures may be well-tolerated and offer healthy probiotics.

Proteins:

Poultry: Skinless poultry, including chicken and turkey, is a lean, low-acid protein source that may be used in meals that are suitable for people with gastritis.

Tofu: Tofu is a plant-based protein alternative that is simple to digest and flexible in preparation.

Beverages:

Water: staying well-hydrated is vital for digestive health, and water is the best option for people with gastritis.

Herbal Teas: Herbal teas like chamomile, peppermint, and ginger may be calming and give hydration without the acidity of caffeinated drinks. Incorporating low-acidity food selections into your diet may go a long way in treating gastritis symptoms and aiding stomach healing.

It's crucial to note that although these meals are typically well-tolerated, individual sensitivities might differ. Therefore, it's essential to maintain a food diary to document your individual triggers and speak with a healthcare practitioner or a qualified dietitian to design a tailored gastritis-friendly meal plan that matches your unique requirements and preferences. With the correct food choices, you may take proactive steps toward alleviating gastritis-related pain and maintaining your overall digestive well-being.

Anti-inflammatory Food Options for Gastritis Management

In the search for successful gastritis treatment, including anti-inflammatory foods in your diet may be a potent technique. Gastritis, characterized by stomach lining inflammation, frequently benefits from a technique that decreases inflammation in the digestive system. Incorporating foods recognized for their anti-inflammatory characteristics may help reduce discomfort and improve stomach healing.

Here, we cover a selection of anti-inflammatory food items that might be helpful additions to your gastritis-friendly diet.

1. Fatty Fish: Fatty fish like salmon, mackerel, and sardines are rich in omega-3 fatty acids, which offer significant anti-inflammatory qualities. These fatty acids may help decrease inflammation in the stomach lining and throughout the digestive tract.

2. Whole Grains: Whole grains such as oats, brown rice, and quinoa are good providers of fiber and minerals. They not only give continuous energy but also help with overall digestive health by lowering inflammation in the stomach.

3. Berries: Blueberries, strawberries, and raspberries are filled with antioxidants, notably anthocyanins, which have anti-inflammatory properties. These fruits may be a delightful and healthy addition to your diet.

4. Leafy greens are full of vitamins, minerals, and phytonutrients that reduce inflammation, such as spinach, kale, and Swiss chard. These

greens may improve the nutritional value of salads and smoothies.

5. Fruits and Vegetables: Almonds, walnuts, flaxseeds, and chia seeds are examples of nuts and seeds that are strong in anti-inflammatory chemicals. They may be eaten as a snack, added to porridge, or sprinkled over yogurt.

6. Turmeric: Curcumin, a potent anti-inflammatory molecule, is a component of the brilliant yellow spice turmeric. Try making turmeric tea or using it in your recipes for its ability to soothe the stomach.

7. Ginger: Another spice with anti-inflammatory and digestive properties is ginger. It may be soaked to make ginger tea or used in both savory and sweet meals.

8. Olive Oil: Monounsaturated fats are abundant in extra-virgin olive oil, which also includes oleocanthal, an ibuprofen-like anti-inflammatory

substance. It makes a wholesome addition to dishes and salad dressings.

9. Green tea: Catechins, an abundant class of antioxidants in green tea, have anti-inflammatory actions. It may be peaceful and healthy to sip on green tea.

10. Berries: Antioxidants are abundant in berries like blueberries, strawberries, and raspberries, especially anthocyanins, which have anti-inflammatory properties. You may include these fruits in your diet as a delightful and wholesome supplement.

11. Garlic: Allicin, a substance having anti-inflammatory and antibacterial effects, is found in garlic. It may be used to provide a variety of food tastes.

12. Avocado: Avocado includes monounsaturated fats and antioxidants that may help decrease inflammation in addition to being creamy and tasty.

These anti-inflammatory food choices may help with symptom alleviation and promote the repair of the stomach lining when included in a gastritis-friendly diet.

It's crucial to keep in mind that everyone reacts to food differently. Consider working with a healthcare practitioner or a qualified dietitian to develop a healthy food plan that is suited to your individual requirements and interests. You may proactively treat gastritis and encourage a healthier, more pleasant digestive tract with the correct anti-inflammatory diet combination.

Foods High in Fiber to Treat Gastritis Dietary fiber is essential for maintaining digestive health, and including fiber-rich foods in one's diet may be especially advantageous for those who suffer from gastritis. Constipation and other digestive problems, such as inflammation of the stomach lining, may result from gastroenteritis. Foods high in fiber may aid in easing such problems and improving overall gut health.

Here, we look at a variety of foods high in fiber that might be beneficial additions to your diet if you have gastritis.

1. Oats: Oats are a flexible, high-fiber food that might be a calming alternative for those with gastritis. Particularly, oatmeal may provide a warm and comfortable breakfast while encouraging gastrointestinal regularity.

2. Brown rice: Compared to white rice, brown rice is a whole grain that has more fiber. It may improve digestion and provide a healthy basis for many different meals.

3. Pasta made using whole wheat: A pasta option that is high in fiber is whole wheat pasta. It may be added to pasta meals and provides the advantage of more nutritional fiber.

4. In addition to being high in fiber and protein, quinoa is a nutrient-dense grain. It tastes well as a main meal, a side dish, or an addition to salads.

5. The legumes Chickpeas, lentils, and beans are great sources of both fiber and protein. They may be used in salads, soups, stews, and other foods as a meat alternative.

6. Fruits are beneficial for digestive health since many of them are rich in dietary fiber. Apples, pears, berries, and citrus fruits (if well tolerated) are among the examples.

7. Broccoli, Brussels sprouts, carrots, and sweet potatoes are fiber-rich vegetables that may be consumed in moderation if you have gastritis.

8. In addition to being providers of good fats, almonds, walnuts, flaxseeds, and chia seeds also include dietary fiber. They may be used as snacks or as an addition to yogurt and oats.

9. Psyllium husk: to improve fiber consumption and encourage regular bowel movements, add psyllium husk, a soluble fiber supplement, to water or smoothies.

10. Chia seeds are an adaptable source of fiber that, after being soaked in liquid, take on the consistency of a gel and may be added to smoothies, puddings, or used to thicken other foods.

11. Spinach: A leafy green that is high in dietary fiber, vitamins, and minerals is spinach. It may be a side dish or added to salads and smoothies.

12. Brussels sprouts, a tasty and wholesome side dish, roasted or steamed Brussels sprouts are a vegetable that is high in fiber. Your gastritis-friendly diet may help to encourage regular digestion, minimize constipation, and support overall stomach health by including these fiber-rich foods.

If you're not used to eating a high-fiber diet, you should introduce fiber gradually since a rapid increase in fiber consumption might sometimes cause stomach pain. Individual tolerances may also differ, so it's best to speak with a medical expert or a trained dietitian to develop a customized gastritis-friendly meal plan that takes into account your particular dietary requirements and preferences.

You may prevent gastritis and enjoy better digestive health by eating the correct balance of fiber-rich foods.

Lean Protein Options for the Treatment of Gastritis: A healthy diet must include protein; however, while controlling gastritis, the choice of protein sources is crucial. Lean protein choices may help lessen the risk of worsening gastritis symptoms and improve digestive pain. A diet that is easy on the stomach often helps people with gastropathy, which is characterized by inflammation of the stomach lining. Here, we look at a variety of lean protein choices that might enhance your meals for those with gastritis.

Chicken without skin: Turkey and skinless chicken are both great sources of lean protein.

Compared to fattier beef or skinless poultry, they are less likely to cause stomach aches. 2. Lean Cuts of Animal Product: Choose lean cuts of beef or pig, such as loin chops, sirloin, or tenderloin. These slices are simpler to digest and have less fat.

Fish: Salmon, mackerel, and trout are examples of fatty fish that are high in protein and omega-3 fatty acids. They not only provide vital nutrients, but they also contain anti-inflammatory qualities that may help with the treatment of gastritis.

Tofu, a soy-based protein, may be used in many meals in place of meat since it is simple to digest. It's a great choice for vegan or vegetarian diets.

Tempeh: Similar to tofu, tempeh is a soy-based protein that has undergone less processing. It is a flexible option for dishes that are suitable for people with gastritis since it has a nutty taste and a hard texture.

Eggs: In addition to being a flexible source of lean protein, eggs may also be boiled, poached, or scrambled. In general, people with gastritis tolerate them well.

Low-Fat Dairy: For individuals who can consume dairy, low-fat choices such as skim milk or plain yogurt may provide protein without the added fat that can cause symptoms.

Legumes: Plant-based protein sources that are rich in fiber and low in fat include beans, lentils, and chickpeas. They may be used in salads, soups, stews, and other dishes.

Seafood: When served without excessive spices, seafood choices like shrimp, crab, and white fish (like cod and haddock), which are normally low in fat, may be pleasant on the stomach.

Seitan, A high-protein meat replacement manufactured from gluten is called seitan, often known as wheat meat or wheat gluten. For individuals seeking substitutes for animal protein made from plants, this is a good choice. It's crucial to pay attention to cooking techniques while choosing and preparing lean protein options for managing gastritis.

The risk of stomach lining irritation may be reduced by using milder cooking methods, including grilling, baking, steaming, and poaching. Individual protein tolerance levels might vary, so it's best to speak with a medical expert or a certified dietitian to develop a custom gastritis meal plan that takes into account your particular dietary requirements and preferences. You may prevent gastritis and boost your overall digestive health by selecting lean protein sources and cooking them in stomach-friendly methods.

Mild and Spicy Foods to Relieve Gastritis

Choosing moderate and non-spicy foods is an important part of the diet for controlling gastritis. Foods that are hot and that have a lot of seasoning may make gastroenteritis, which is characterized by inflammation of the stomach lining, worse. It's crucial to choose softer, gentler solutions to decrease pain and the possibility of bringing on symptoms of gastritis. Here, we look at a selection of mild and unseasoned foods that might be calming and helpful for those who have gastritis.

1. Congee or plain rice: For those with gastritis, a simple bowl of plain steamed rice or rice congee (rice porridge) might be soothing and straightforward to digest.

2. Bland Pasta: A mild and satisfying supper may be made from pasta dishes with little flavor, including plain spaghetti with olive oil or a simple garlic and herb sauce.

3. Mashable potatoes: Using low-fat milk or butter to make creamy mashed potatoes may make for a filling and relaxing side dish.

4. Steamed Vegetables: When served without excessive flavors, steamed vegetables like carrots, zucchini, or green beans are gentle on

the stomach. Herbs and a splash of olive oil may be used to enhance flavor.

5. Grilled or poached chicken: Poached or simply grilled skinless, boneless chicken breast may provide a lean protein supply without the discomfort that may result with fried or highly spicy dishes.

6. White Fish: Mild white fish, such as cod or tilapia, may be served delicately and with little spice, making it acceptable for those with gastritis.

7. Broiled or baked tofu: Tofu may be used as a plant-based protein substitute for bland foods when baked or grilled with a little marinade or soy sauce.

8. Oatmeal: Oatmeal may be a calming breakfast or snack when it's cooked with water or low-fat milk and sweetened with a little honey or mashed banana. Greek yogurt that is unflavored

9. Plain Greek yogurt is a low-fat and probiotic-rich choice that tastes great when paired with fresh, non-acidic fruit or drizzled with honey.

10. Rice Cakes with Nut Butter, number ten Rice cakes are a filling and simple-to-digest snack choice that may be smeared with almond or peanut butter (if permitted).

11. Vegetable Soup: A homemade vegetable soup cooked using non-spicy veggies and a moderate broth may be nourishing and comforting.

12. Eggs and Scrambles: A mild and protein-rich breakfast or supper may be produced with scrambled eggs that have little spice and are served with bread on the side.

Keep seasoning to a minimum and stay away from components that are known to exacerbate symptoms while making mild and spicy foods for the alleviation of gastritis. These include hot sauces, spicy peppers, and excessively spiced condiments.

Additionally, healthier alternatives to frying or deep-frying include steaming, boiling, baking, or grilling. To develop a customized gastritis-friendly meal plan that meets your individual dietary requirements and preferences, it is advised to speak with a healthcare provider or a qualified dietitian. Individual tolerances for certain foods may differ.

You may actively manage gastritis and take pleasure in meals that are soothing and beneficial to your digestive health by selecting moderate and non-spicy selections.

Adaptogenic Drinks for Soothing Relief from Gastritis

For those who are treating gastritis, selecting the proper beverages is crucial since certain drinks either reduce or increase symptoms. Gastritis, which is characterized by stomach lining inflammation, often necessitates the consumption of mild, calming drinks that won't irritate the sensitive gastric tissues. Here, we look at a variety of mild drinks that are good for people with gastritis and may help with pain management and digestive healing.

1. Water: For intestinal health, it's essential to stay hydrated. The ideal option is plain water since it keeps you hydrated overall without irritating your stomach.

2. Herbal teas: Teas made from herbs may be quite calming for gastritis.

Several mild choices include:

Tea made from chamomile: Chamomile tea, which has soothing and anti-inflammatory qualities, helps ease the symptoms of gastritis.

Tea with peppermint flavor: Although peppermint tea might be potent for some people, it can also aid with indigestion and stomach pain if drank in moderation.

Ginger tea, Ginger may help with digestion and have anti-inflammatory qualities. A calming option for gastritis treatment is ginger tea.

3. Licorice Root Tea: Deglycyrrhizinated licorice (DGL), which is used to make licorice root tea, has anti-inflammatory and pain-relieving properties.

4. Aloe vera juice, when eaten in moderation and without additional sweets, may have calming effects on the stomach lining.

5. Coconut Water: Coconut water is a stomach-friendly and hydrated choice that is often well-tolerated.

6. Rice water, the starchy liquid that remains after boiling rice, is a bland and calming beverage option.

7. Almond milk: For those with lactose sensitivity, unsweetened almond milk may be used in lieu of ordinary milk since it is dairy-free.

8. Non-Citrus Fruit Juices: Citrus liquids should be avoided because of their high acidity; however, non-citrus fruit juices like apple or pear juice may be more palatable. Smoothies made with plain yogurt

9. Smoothies produced with non-acidic fruits like bananas and plain yogurt, ideally low-fat, may provide nutrients and probiotics without causing discomfort.

10. Teas and coffees without caffeine: If you like tea or coffee, choosing decaffeinated varieties may help lower the possibility of triggering too much stomach acid.

11. Bone Broth: Bone broth is mild on the stomach and may deliver minerals that assist digestive health. Individual tolerances can vary,

so it's best to pay attention to how your body reacts to these drinks and seek advice from a medical professional or registered dietitian for dietary recommendations that are tailored to your particular case of gastritis severity and underlying causes.

[You may also want to check out my fantastic cookbook on the Bone Broth Diet, The Wonder Bone Broth Diet Cookbook by Lydia G. Perez, and explore the awesome diets that can not only aid in healing gastritis but also other amazing health benefits]

You may take proactive steps to control your disease, reduce pain, and encourage stomach healing by choosing mild gastritis-friendly drinks. Additionally, you must limit or completely avoid alcoholic beverages, carbonated drinks, and highly caffeinated beverages from your diet since they might aggravate the symptoms of gastritis.

Ingredients that are Good for Gastritis for Digestive Comfort

The selection of components is just as important when creating a diet that is conducive to gastritis as the choice of certain meals. When treating gastropathy, which is characterized by inflammation of the stomach lining, it's important to concentrate on using calming, mild medicines. By being aware of the foods that work best for managing gastritis, you may prepare meals that support gastrointestinal comfort and encourage stomach healing.

Here, we look at a variety of components that are suitable for dishes if you have gastritis.

1. Plain Rice: Plain white or brown rice is a flexible component that may be used as a basis for a variety of cuisines that are suitable for people with gastritis.

2. Oats: Oats may be used to produce oatmeal and provide soluble fiber for digestive health, whether they are rolled oats or steel-cut oats.

3. Healthy Proteins: Skinless Poultry: Lean protein sources that may be utilized in a variety of cuisines include chicken and turkey breast. Fish: When served with a little spice, mild white fish like cod or tilapia is easy on the stomach. Tofu is a flexible plant-based protein that may be used in a variety of dishes.

4. Fruits That Aren't Acidic:

Bananas: Bananas are a calming and readily digested fruit that may be eaten as a snack or as an addition to smoothies.

Apples may be added to salads or used as a topping for oatmeal since they have a low acidity.

5. Citrus-Free Vegetables:

Carrots: A non-acidic vegetable, carrots may be utilized in a variety of cooked and raw dishes.

Spinach: Spinach is a nutrient-dense leafy green that is often well-tolerated.

6. Whole Grains: Substances such as quinoa, whole wheat pasta, and whole grain bread may provide fiber and crucial nutrients.

7. Low-Fat Dairy or Dairy Alternatives: Those who can consume dairy products may choose lactose-free milk or plain yogurt as low-fat substitutes. For those with lactose sensitivity, non-dairy options like soy yogurt or almond milk are acceptable.

8. Mild Herbs and Spices: Some mild herbs and spices that might help with gastritis include:

Ginger: Known for its ability to reduce inflammation, ginger may be used to season food or to produce a calming ginger tea.

Turmeric: Curcumin, an anti-inflammatory chemical, is present in turmeric. It may be converted into a golden milk beverage or used to season a variety of meals.

Fennel: Fennel seeds or fresh fennel may give food a mild, comforting taste.

9. Olive oil and coconut oil are moderate cooking and salad dressing oils that may be utilized.

10. Low-sodium chicken or vegetable broths may be used as the foundation for soups and stews.

11. Rice Cakes: An unappetizing and tasteless snack choice are rice cakes.

15. Choose lean ground meat like turkey or chicken if you choose to have meat in your diet. They may be included in a variety of dishes, including casseroles, stir-fries, and soups.

16. Eggs are an adaptable and simple-to-digest source of protein. An easy dinner choice would be eggs—scrambled, boiled, or in omelets—with non-acidic veggies.

17. Consider low-FODMAP components like rice, gluten-free oats, lactose-free dairy, and certain fruits and vegetables like spinach and zucchini if you have gastritis that is brought on by certain fermentable carbs (FODMAPs).

18. Almonds, walnuts, sunflower seeds, and pumpkin seeds are just a few of the nuts and seeds that may be added to yogurt, oats, or smoothies to give them more texture and nutrition.

19. Mild Cheeses: Some people with gastritis may have mild cheeses like cottage cheese or mozzarella. To add taste and protein, use them in moderation.

20. Fresh herbs, such as basil, parsley, and cilantro, may infuse foods with flavor without irritating the palate.

21. Low-Acidity Vinegars: While some people may have issues with vinegar, dressings or marinades may be made using low-acidity vinegars such as rice vinegar or apple cider vinegar (when used sparingly).

22. Nut Butters: Nut butters, such as almond or cashew butter, are nutrient-dense and may be used in smoothies or spread over rice cakes (if permitted).

23. Non-Alcoholic Bitters: Using non-alcoholic bitters before meals might help some people with the symptoms of gastritis. These may be applied as needed and in moderation.

Keep an eye on portion proportions since overeating, even with mild components, might strain the stomach more. Also, take into account any dietary sensitivities or limits you may have, since they might differ from person to person. Utilizing these foods calls for an emphasis on simplicity while avoiding excessively processed items, strong spices, and acidic chemicals. Consult with a healthcare expert or a qualified dietitian who can assist you in developing a customized gastritis-friendly meal plan to make sure your dietary decisions are in line with your specific requirements and tastes.

Investigating Natural Remedies for Gastritis

Certain nutrients have therapeutic characteristics that may help reduce inflammation, promote digestive comfort, and encourage stomach repair while treating gastritis. A gastritis-friendly diet that emphasizes these therapeutic foods is beneficial for treating the condition of gastroenteritis, which is characterized by inflammation of the stomach lining. We'll look at a few of these foods that may improve your meals in this article.

1. Honey: Honey is well-known for its calming effects and may help coat the stomach lining, offering alleviation from the pain associated with gastritis. As a natural sweetener, use raw, unprocessed honey and use it sparingly.

2. Aloe vera may provide calming and anti-inflammatory effects on the stomach lining when ingested as juice (without additional sweeteners or laxatives).

3. Deglycyrrhizinated licorice (DGL), a kind of licorice root, may help preserve the stomach lining and relieve the symptoms of gastritis. It is often offered as a chewable tablet or as a dietary supplement.

4. Marshmallow Root: Mucilaginous marshmallow root has the ability to establish a layer of defense around the stomach lining. It is often sold as a tea or dietary supplement.

5. Like marshmallow root, slippery elm contains mucilage that helps calm and shield the stomach

lining. Usually, it comes in the form of a powdered supplement or tea.

6. Bone Broth: Homemade bone broth is a great source of collagen and amino acids, which promote digestive health and may even help the stomach lining recover.

[You may also want to check out my fantastic cookbook on the Bone Broth Diet, The Wonder Bone Broth Diet Cookbook by Lydia G. Perez, and explore the awesome diets that can not only aid in healing gastritis but also other amazing health benefits]

7. Fresh cabbage juice, which may have anti-inflammatory and therapeutic effects, has been shown to help some people with gastritis.

8. Foods that are high in probiotics include yogurt, kefir, and sauerkraut. Probiotics may help maintain a healthy gut microbiota and may even help treat gastritis.

9. Papaya: Papaya includes digestive enzymes like papain that may also be able to calm the stomach.

10. Manuka Honey: Manuka honey is a unique kind of honey from New Zealand that may have antibacterial effects. It should only be taken sparingly for maximum benefit.

11. Boneless, skinless chicken broth: Boneless, skinless chicken broth may be soothing to the stomach and nourishing.

12. Non-Alcoholic Ginger Beer: Some people find that drinking non-alcoholic ginger beer helps to alleviate the symptoms of gastritis. Ginger is well-known for reducing inflammation.

13. Chamomile: Due to its possible sedative properties, chamomile may be used in food preparations in addition to being sold as tea.

14. Banana: Bananas are naturally occurring, non-acidic fruits that might provide a source of fiber and energy while also perhaps calming the stomach.

15. Mastic Gum: Mastic gum, a resin from the mastic tree, is sold as a supplement and is said to have stomach-soothing qualities.

It's important to keep in mind that different people may respond differently to these therapeutic elements, even though they may provide comfort and support for gastritis. They should not be used as the only form of therapy for gastritis; rather, they should be a component of a well-balanced diet. To make sure these substances are safely included in your diet and that they meet your specific requirements and preferences related to your gastritis, it is advised to speak with a healthcare provider or a qualified dietitian.

You may actively participate in the treatment of your gastritis and encourage comfort and healing for the stomach by learning more about these restorative components.

Gastritis-Specific Ingredients Included for Targeted Relief

It's crucial to take into account components that are recognized for their advantages in treating gastritis while dealing with the ailment. Gastritis, which is characterized by inflammation of the stomach lining, often necessitates the use of foods that might reduce symptoms and hasten recovery.

Here, we look at a few foods that are specifically designed to treat gastritis and may be added to meals for targeted relief and better digestive health.

1. Foods high in fiber: Dietary fiber may help calm and protect the stomach lining. Think of including these high-fiber components:

Oats: A mild and high-fiber option is oatmeal cooked with water or low-fat milk. Brown rice: Brown rice is a complete grain that contains healthy fiber. Bananas: In addition to being simple to digest, bananas also contain soluble fiber.

2. Ginger: Ginger's anti-inflammatory qualities are widely recognized, and it may aid with stomach pain. Include ginger in a variety of forms.

Ginger Tea: Steep fresh ginger slices in hot water to make a calming cup of ginger tea.

Ginger in Cooking: For more flavor and maybe some relief, use fresh ginger in your meals.

3. Curcumin, which is found in turmeric, has anti-inflammatory effects.

Here is how to apply it:

Turmeric Milk (Golden Milk): Combine milk, turmeric, and a dash of black pepper to make a warm beverage. Add turmeric to your favorite curries and stews for taste and maybe to help with gastritis.

4. Aloe Vera: When drunk in moderation without additional sweets, aloe vera juice may have calming effects on the stomach lining.

5. Fennel: Fennel seeds or fresh fennel bulbs may give your dishes a calming, licorice-like taste and perhaps help with digestion.

6. Foods High in Probiotics: Probiotics have been shown to support a healthy gut flora and may be helpful for gastritis.

Take into account:

Yogurt with Live Microorganisms: Select plain yogurt that has live probiotic microorganisms.

Kefir: Kefir is a probiotic-rich fermented dairy product.

Sauerkraut: Sauerkraut is a kind of fermented food that contains probiotics.

7. Mint: Mint has the potential to ease indigestion and ease stomach pain.

It may be used for the following uses:

Peppermint tea: make a relaxing cup of peppermint tea.

Fresh Peppermint Leaves: Infuse water with fresh peppermint leaves or add them to salads.

8. Manuka Honey: Manuka honey may be used as a natural sweetener in moderation and is renowned for its possible antibacterial capabilities.

9. Deglycyrrhizinated licorice (DGL), a dietary supplement made from licorice root, may aid in protecting the stomach lining.

10. Marshmallow root includes mucilage, which may calm the stomach lining and is available as a supplement or tea.

11. Papaya: Papaya has enzymes, such as papain, that may help with digestion and provide comfort.

Make sure your entire meal plan is balanced and well-suited to your unique requirements and tastes when using these gastritis-specific items in your diet. Individual tolerances might vary, so talk to a trained dietitian or healthcare provider to develop a custom, gastritis-friendly diet that takes into account your particular situation.

You may actively work toward treating gastritis symptoms and promoting stomach comfort and healing by adding these particular substances. *The Function of Probiotics in the Treatment of*

Gastritis Probiotics, sometimes known as "good" or "friendly" bacteria, are important for preserving gut health and may be helpful for those with gastritis. Gastritis, which is characterized by stomach lining inflammation, may upset the harmony of the gut microbiome, which is made up of a range of bacteria that affect digestion and general health.

Here, we examine the function of probiotics in the treatment of gastritis and how they might promote healing and comfort for the digestive system.

1. Restoring Gut Microbiome Balance: Gastritis has the potential to change the makeup of the gut microbiome, which might result in an increase in dangerous bacteria or a decrease in good ones. Regular use of probiotics may aid in reestablishing this equilibrium by introducing healthy bacteria into the digestive tract. These "friendly" bacteria may outcompete unfavorable types, perhaps lowering inflammation and promoting the health of the stomach.

2. Increasing Digestive Function: Probiotics may help with nutrition absorption and digestion. They help the body digest food, especially complex carbohydrates, and aid in the body's ability to absorb vital vitamins and minerals from the diet. The burden on the stomach may be lessened, and comfort can be increased by this enhanced digestion.

3. Gut Lining Stabilization: Some probiotic strains have been demonstrated to stabilize the intestinal barrier, which is advantageous for those who have gastritis. A gut lining that is stronger and healthier may be less prone to irritation and inflammation.

4. Reducing Inflammation: Some probiotics are anti-inflammatory. They could aid in reducing gastritis symptoms and promoting the healing process by reducing general inflammation in the gut.

5. Support for the Immune System: The gut is home to a significant percentage of the immune system, and a healthy gut flora is necessary for a robust immune system. Probiotics may help maintain this equilibrium, perhaps improving the body's capacity to fight off infections or other pathogens that could aggravate gastritis.

6. Bloating, gas, and irregular bowel movements are among the symptoms that some people with gastritis encounter. By encouraging a more streamlined and regular digestive process, probiotics may be able to reduce these symptoms. It's important to choose the correct probiotic strains and products when contemplating probiotics for the treatment of gastritis. Probiotics are not all created equal, and the strains that are employed might affect their efficacy.

The probiotic bacteria Lactobacillus and Bifidobacterium are two popular ones that may be helpful for gastritis. When utilizing probiotics for gastritis, keep the following things in mind:

Consult with a Healthcare Professional: Before beginning any new supplement, including probiotics, speak with a medical expert or a certified dietitian who can provide advice based on your specific health issues and requirements.

Choose trustworthy brands that list the strain(s) and colony-forming units (CFUs) per dosage if you decide to take probiotic supplements.

Dietary Sources: Fermented foods including yogurt, kefir, sauerkraut, and kimchi are also good sources of probiotics. These items may be included in a healthy, gastritis-friendly diet as a natural source of probiotics.

Consistency: Probiotics work best when consumed regularly over time. It could take a few weeks before the symptoms of gastritis start to get better.

Monitor for Tolerance: Keep an eye on your body's reaction to probiotics. If you encounter any negative effects or a worsening of your symptoms, stop using the medication and seek medical advice.

In conclusion, by encouraging a healthy gut flora, lowering inflammation, and supporting digestive comfort and healing, probiotics may be a useful part of gastritis care. To make sure that they work with your unique case of gastritis and dietary preferences, their usage should be handled with advice from a medical specialist.

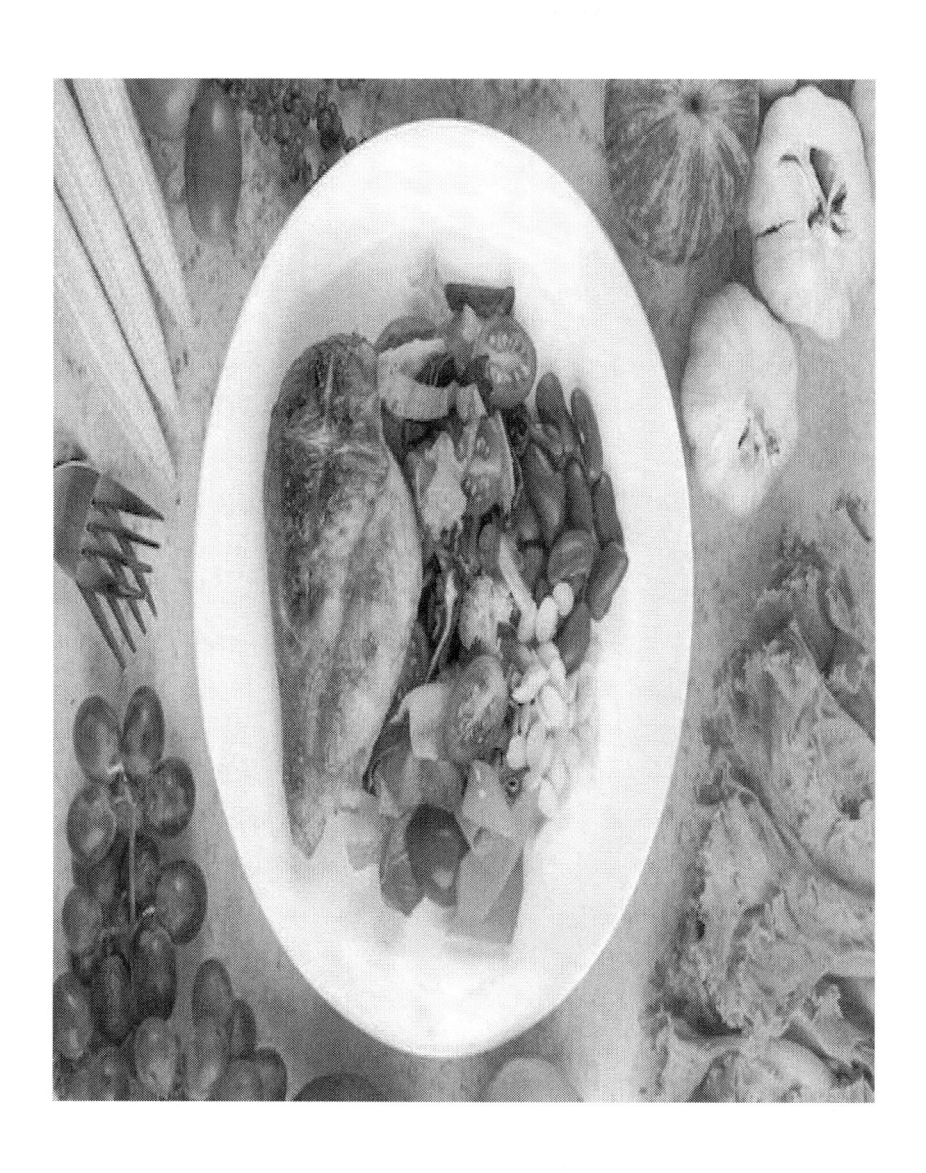

CHAPTER TWO

Meal Planning and Sample Menus for Gastritis

Key Considerations for Meal Preparation for Gastritis Careful selection of meals and components is essential when meal planning for those with gastritis in order to lessen symptoms, calm inflammation, and encourage healing of the stomach. When preparing meals for gastritis, keep the following points in mind:

1. Small, Repeated Meals Reduce the chance of discomfort by choosing smaller, more frequent meals throughout the day. This will prevent the stomach from becoming overloaded. This may promote digestion and help keep blood sugar levels constant.

2. Blank and Unsuccessful: To prevent the lining of the stomach from being irritated, choose moderate and unseasoned meals. Steer clear of

strong flavors, spicy foods, and acidic components.

3. Balanced Diet: Strive to eat a diet that is composed of a range of food categories. This guarantees that you get the nutrients you need and supports general health.

4. Hydration: Drink plenty of simple water or mild drinks like herbal teas to stay hydrated. Drinks with caffeine and carbonation should be avoided since they might irritate the stomach.

5. Probiotics: To promote gut health and lower inflammation, think about including probiotic-rich meals or supplements.

6. Avoid foods that aggravate your gastritis symptoms by identifying them. These may vary from person to person but often include fatty, spicy, and acidic meals.

7. Portion Control: Watch your portion proportions to prevent overeating, which may strain your stomach even more.

8. Meal Timing: To lower the chance of acid reflux and discomfort when lying down, give yourself at least two to three hours between meals and at night.

Here are three example menus for breakfast, lunch, and supper to help you with meal planning:

Breakfast Sample Menu for Gastritis:

Oatmeal: Prepared with low-fat milk or water and garnished with sliced bananas and honey. Ginger Tea: Warm, unsweetened ginger tea might help settle the stomach.

Scrambled Eggs: A little serving of eggs scrambled with a little spice.

Lunch Sample Menu for Gastritis:

Grilled Chicken Salad: A skinless, boneless chicken breast that has been lightly seasoned and grilled is served over a bed of mixed greens (lettuce, spinach), with cucumber slices and a straightforward olive oil and lemon dressing. A modest serving of plain, steamed rice is served on the side.

Greek yogurt, served plain and garnished with ground flaxseeds, in a small portion Dinner

Menu Example for Gastritis

Mild white fish, such as cod or tilapia, is cooked with a little olive oil and fresh herbs (such as rosemary or dill).

Mashed Potatoes: Rich, creamy mashed potatoes cooked with lactose-free milk or a little bit of butter.

Steamed Vegetables: Green beans and carrots served steamed.

Chamomile tea: Before going to bed, sip on a relaxing cup of chamomile tea.

--- Though individual tastes and tolerances may differ, these example menus provide suggestions for meals that are suitable for people with gastritis. Customizing your meal plan to meet your unique nutritional requirements is crucial. For individualized advice, speak with a healthcare provider or registered dietitian.

To successfully treat gastritis, keep in mind the significance of portion management and avoiding trigger foods. A monthly meal plan for a gastritis diet must be varied, and each meal must be easy on the stomach. To get you started, here is an example monthly food plan. As individual tolerances and tastes might differ, feel free to modify as necessary to meet your requirements.

Week 1:

Day 1: Oatmeal with sliced bananas and a dab of honey for breakfast.

Steamed rice and mixed greens with grilled chicken breast for lunch

For dinner, steaming vegetables and mashed potatoes with baked white fish

Greek yogurt in its purest form

Day 2: Breakfast on the second day was scrambled eggs with some plain bread.

Quinoa salad with bell peppers, cucumber, and a mild olive oil dressing for lunch

Stir-fried turkey and vegetables with brown rice for dinner

apple slices as a snack.

Day 3: Greek yogurt with ground flaxseeds and a dab of honey for breakfast

Lunch: Plain rice cakes and lentil soup.

baked fish, roasted sweet potatoes, and steamed broccoli for dinner.

rice pudding prepared with lactose-free milk as a snack.

Day 4: A smoothie prepared with banana, spinach, and unsweetened almond milk for breakfast

Use a whole-grain tortilla for the spinach and a grilled chicken wrap for lunch.

Tofu stir-fry with bok choy and brown rice for dinner

Sliced cucumbers as a snack

Day 5: Breakfast on the fifth day was rice congee with diced chicken and a hint of ginger.

Quinoa and black bean salad with a simple vinaigrette dressing for lunch

Roasted turkey breast served with mashed sweet potatoes and steaming green beans for dinner

Snack: fruit salad without citrus (such as melons and berries).

Day 6: Breakfast was poached eggs and steamed spinach.

rice, chicken, and vegetable soup for lunch.

Grilled shrimp with quinoa and asparagus for dinner

Greek yogurt with a dash of cinnamon as a snack

Day 7: Oat bran cereal with almond milk and sliced peaches for breakfast

whole-grain bread with a turkey and avocado sandwich for lunch.

Dinner will consist of baked fish, mashed cauliflower, and sautéed spinach.

a handful of unsalted almonds as a snack.

Week 2

Day 1: For breakfast, combine plain Greek yogurt with ripe banana slices and a dash of flaxseed meal.

Grilled chicken breast served with quinoa and steamed broccoli for lunch

white fish baked in the oven with mashed sweet potatoes and sautéed spinach for dinner.

rice cakes with almond butter as a snack.

Day 2:

Breakfast: Oatmeal prepared with lactose-free milk or water and garnished with sliced strawberries and honey.

Lunch: Plain rice cakes and lentil and vegetable soup.

Dinner: brown rice and turkey stir-fry with bell peppers and zucchini.

Snack: Melon slices.

Day 3:

For breakfast, scrambled eggs with fresh basil and chopped tomatoes

Spinach and grilled chicken salad with a mild lemon and olive oil dressing for lunch

Salmon was baked in the oven with quinoa and steamed asparagus for dinner.

Snack: fruit salad that isn't citrus (such as grapes and kiwis).

Day 4:

Smoothie with banana, spinach, and unsweetened almond milk for breakfast

whole-grain tortilla wrapped around turkey and avocado for lunch.

tofu, veggie, and brown rice stir-fry for dinner.

Snack: Plain yogurt on the side with slices of cucumber.

Day 5:

Rice congee with chicken shreds and a hint of grated ginger for breakfast.

Quinoa and black bean salad with a simple vinaigrette dressing for lunch

Roasted turkey breast, mashed butternut squash, and steaming green beans for dinner

a handful of unsalted almonds as a snack.

Day 6:

Poached eggs with sautéed spinach for breakfast

plain rice and chicken-and-vegetable soup for lunch.

Grilled shrimp with quinoa and sautéed bok cabbage for dinner

peach slices as a snack.

Day 7:

Oat bran cereal with almond milk and fresh blueberries for breakfast

whole-grain bread with a turkey and cucumber sandwich for lunch.

Baked fish with mashed cauliflower and steamed vegetables for dinner

a snack of hummus and rice cakes.

Week 3

Day 1:

For breakfast, have scrambled eggs, sautéed spinach, and whole-wheat bread.

Quinoa with grilled chicken and vegetables for lunch

For dinner, steaming green beans and roasted sweet potatoes will be served with baked fish.

a small handful of unsalted almonds for a snack.

Day 2:

Greek yogurt parfait with fresh berry and honey layers for breakfast

mixed green salad and lentil and vegetable soup for lunch.

Stir-fried turkey and vegetables with brown rice for dinner

Snack: Hummus and cucumber slices.

Day 3:

Smoothie with banana, kale, and unsweetened almond milk for breakfast

Use a whole-grain tortilla for the spinach and a grilled chicken wrap for lunch.

Salmon baked in the oven with quinoa and steamed asparagus for dinner

Snack: fruit salad without citrus (such as melons and grapes).

Day 4:

Breakfast: Oatmeal prepared with lactose-free milk or water and garnished with sliced peaches

Chia seeds whole-grain bread with a turkey and avocado sandwich for lunch.

Tofu, veggie, and quinoa stir-fry for dinner.

Rice cakes with almond butter as a snack.

Day 5:

Rice congee with chicken shreds and a hint of grated ginger for breakfast

Quinoa and black bean salad with a simple vinaigrette dressing for lunch

Shrimp on the grill with mashed sweet potatoes and steamed broccoli for dinner

Snack: A small dish of unsweetened dry fruit and mixed almonds.

Day 6:

Poached eggs with sliced tomatoes and fresh basil for breakfast

plain rice cakes and chicken and vegetable soup for lunch.

White fish was baked in the oven with mashed cauliflower and sauteed spinach for dinner.

Snack: Greek yogurt topped with sliced strawberries.

Day 7:

Oat bran cereal with almond milk and fresh raspberries for breakfast

Lemon-tahini dressing on a mixed greens salad with grilled chicken breast for lunch.

For dinner, roast bell peppers and spaghetti squash with baked turkey meatballs.

Rice cakes with cottage cheese as a snack

Week 4

Day 1:

For breakfast, have scrambled eggs, sautéed spinach, and whole-wheat bread.

Quinoa with grilled chicken and vegetables for lunch

For dinner, steaming green beans and roasted sweet potatoes will be served with baked fish.

A small handful of unsalted almonds for a snack.

Day 2:

Greek yogurt parfait with fresh berry and honey layers for breakfast.

Mixed green salad and lentil and vegetable soup for lunch.

Stir-fried turkey and vegetables with brown rice for dinner

Snack: Hummus and cucumber slices.

Day 3:

Smoothie with banana, kale, and unsweetened almond milk for breakfast

Use a whole-grain tortilla for the spinach and a grilled chicken wrap for lunch.

Salmon baked in the oven with quinoa and steamed asparagus for dinner

Snack: fruit salad without citrus (such as melons and grapes).

Day 4:

Breakfast: Oatmeal prepared with lactose-free milk or water and garnished with sliced peaches

Chia seeds. whole-grain bread with a turkey and avocado sandwich for lunch.

Tofu, veggie, and quinoa stir-fry for dinner.

Rice cakes with almond butter as a snack.

Day 5:

Rice congee with chicken shreds and a hint of grated ginger for breakfast

Quinoa and black bean salad with a simple vinaigrette dressing for lunch

Shrimp on the grill with mashed sweet potatoes and steamed broccoli for dinner

Snack: A small dish of unsweetened dry fruit and mixed almonds.

Day 6:

Poached eggs with sliced tomatoes and fresh basil for breakfast

Plain rice cakes and chicken and vegetable soup for lunch.

White fish was baked in the oven with mashed cauliflower and sauteed spinach for dinner.

Snack: Greek yogurt topped with sliced strawberries.

Day 7:

Oat bran cereal with almond milk and fresh raspberries for breakfast

lemon-tahini dressing on a mixed greens salad with grilled chicken breast for lunch.

For dinner, roast bell peppers and spaghetti squash with baked turkey meatballs.

Rice cakes with cottage cheese as a snack.

As usual, modify it to suit your tastes and dietary requirements. It's still important to stay hydrated with simple water or calming herbal teas, and speaking with a medical practitioner or certified nutritionist for specific advice is advised.

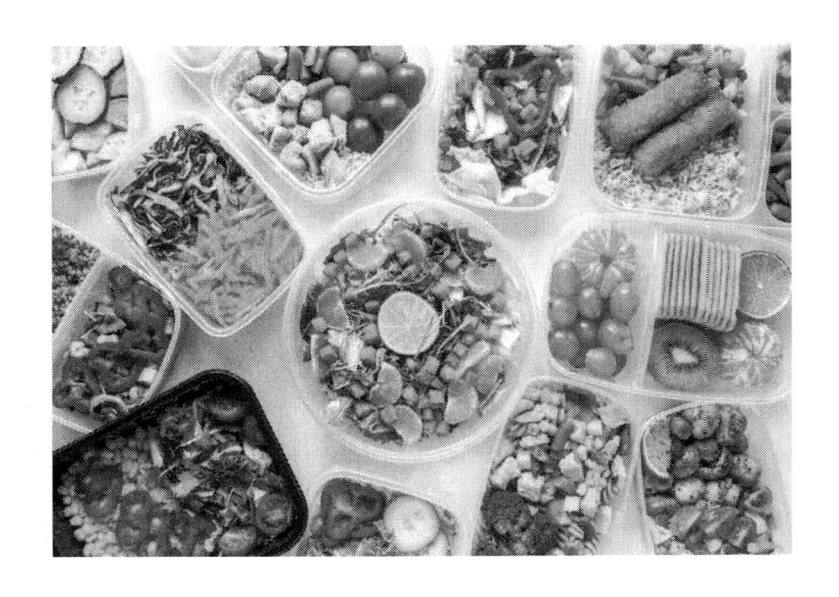

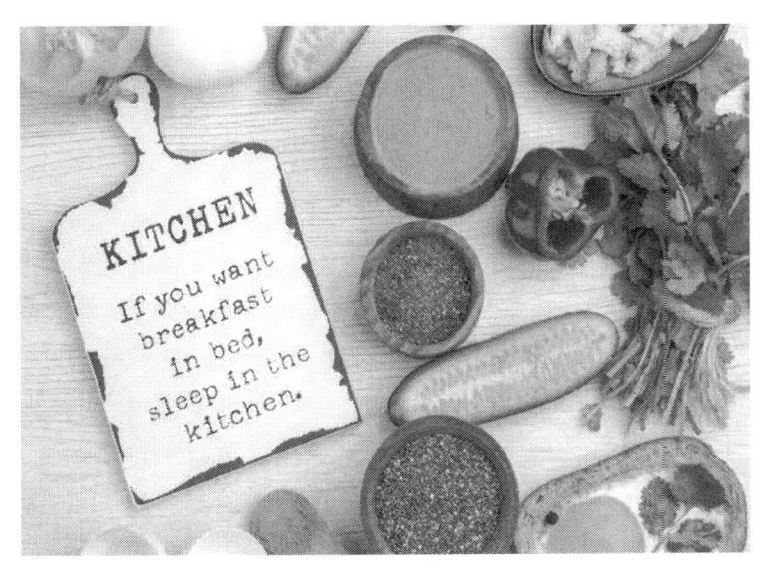

CHAPTER THREE

Cooking Tips and Techniques

To guarantee that meals are soft on the stomach while maintaining taste and nutrients, cooking for gastritis necessitates certain changes. Here are some approaches and culinary hints to help you make meals that are suitable for those with gastritis:

1. Choose between steaming and boiling: Boiling and steaming are moderate cooking techniques that may help foods maintain moisture and nutrients. Think of cooking rice or pasta and steaming veggies.

2. Poaching Protein: You may give chicken, fish, or tofu a flavor boost by poaching them in a tasty broth without adding extra oil or seasonings that could upset your stomach.

3. Minimally Fatty: Sautéing or pan-frying should only require a small quantity of oil or butter. To avoid the need for additional fats, think about non-stick cookware.

4. Lean proteins Pick lean meats like skinless fowl, skinless turkey, and lean beef or pork chops. To make the food simpler to digest, remove any obvious fat.

5. Avoid High Heat: Cooking with high heat, such as grilling or broiling, might result in burnt and perhaps irritable food. Choose low-heat cooking methods.

6. Combining Soups: Without using heavy creams or butter, soups may have a creamy texture by being pureed. This is wonderful for traditional soups that are gastritis-friendly.

7. Herbal tinctures: To give food taste, add mild herbs like basil, oregano, or thyme. Avoid using strong spices and flavors.

8. Homemade broths: Use mild veggies like potatoes, celery, and carrots to make your own broth. For more flavor, simmer them with a little pork or chicken.

9. Gentle Seasonings: Try using spices that have anti-inflammatory effects and may subtly flavor your food, such as ginger and turmeric.

10. Fresh components: Utilize fresh, complete foods wherever feasible. They often have fewer ingredients and are more palatable.

11. Prepare smaller portions to prevent overeating, which may put additional strain on your stomach.

12. Chewing Properly: Give your meal a good, long chew. This facilitates digestion and lowers the possibility of pain.

13. Desserts with less sugar: If you have a sweet craving, choose sweets like fruit salad or rice

pudding prepared with lactose-free milk that are low in sugar or naturally sweetened.

14. Hydroponics: Use calming herbal teas or simple water to stay hydrated. Do not drink anything with carbonation or caffeine.

15. Dietary Fiber: To encourage normal digestion, gradually increase the amount of fiber you consume from fruits, vegetables, and whole grains.

16. Maintain a regular eating pattern with short, frequent meals and avoid missing meals.

17. Keep a food journal to keep note of the meals that make you feel ill so you can avoid them in the future.

18. Speak with a dietitian. Consult a qualified dietitian for individualized advice and meal planning so you can design a diet specifically for your requirements if you have gastritis.

Keep in mind that each person may have a different tolerance for various meals and cooking methods, so it's important to pay attention to your body and modify your cooking techniques and ingredient selections as necessary. The objective is to prepare scrumptious and calming meals that assist your control of gastritis and encourage digestive comfort.

Techniques and Tips for Cooking a Gastritis-Friendly Diet

Gastritis may be a difficult ailment to manage, but with some mindful modifications to your cooking methods and ingredient selections, you can make tasty and calming meals that help your overall wellbeing and improve digestive comfort.

Here, we go into further detail about cooking advice and methods for a gastritis-friendly diet to provide you with a thorough guide to successful cooking while putting stomach health first.

1. Gentle Cooking Techniques: Cooking for those with gastroenteritis begins with selecting moderate techniques that maintain the moisture and nutrients in your foods. Vegetables, cereals, and proteins all benefit greatly from steaming and boiling. By using these techniques, the demand for additional fats is reduced, making food simpler to digest.

2. The Practice of Poaching: Foods are poached by slowly cooking them in a delicious liquid, often a broth. This method adds flavor to proteins like chicken, fish, or tofu without using a lot of extra fats or spices that could irritate the lining of the stomach.

3. Conscious Fat Use: While fats may enhance the taste and richness of your food, they should only be used in moderation in a diet that is conducive to gastritis. When sautéing or pan-frying, use modest quantities of butter,

coconut oil, or olive oil. The requirement for extra fats may be lessened with the use of non-stick cookware.

4. Options for Lean Protein: Choose lean meats such as skinless fowl, skinless turkey, and lean beef or pork. Trim away any obvious fat to reduce the amount that might irritate.

5. Lower Heat Cooking: Foods cooked at high temperatures, such as when grilling or broiling, may become scorched and possibly irritable. Select cooking methods that use less heat, such as baking, simmering, or slow cooking.

6. Velvety soups that are blended: Without using heavy creams or butter, you may still have creamy soups. To generate a smooth texture that is easy on the stomach, just purée your soups.

7. Homemade broths include: Use mild veggies like potatoes, celery, and carrots to make your own broth. For more flavor, simmer them with a little pork or chicken. Broths produced at home

give you more control over the contents and lessen the chance of irritating additives.

8. The Strength of Gentle Spices: Try using spices that may reduce inflammation and give your food a mild taste. Explore ginger, turmeric, and fennel as potential alternatives.

9. Fresh and complete ingredients Utilize fresh, complete foods wherever feasible. They are less likely to have chemicals that might cause symptoms of gastritis. Fresh vegetables are also usually easier on the stomach.

10. Portion Control: To prevent overeating, which may put unneeded strain on your stomach, prepare smaller portion sizes. More frequent, smaller meals may improve digestion and reduce pain.

11. Chew your meal fully: Give your meal a good, long chew. By breaking down food into smaller, more digestible pieces, proper chewing helps with digestion.

12. Desserts with less sugar If you have a sweet craving, choose treats that are naturally sweetened or low in sugar. Satisfying alternatives include fruit salads, rice pudding cooked with lactose-free milk, or baked apples with cinnamon.

13. Remain hydrated: In order to maintain general health and digestive comfort, one must drink enough water. Stay away from fizzy or caffeine-containing drinks that might upset your stomach and instead stick to simple water and relaxing herbal teas.

14. Gradual Fiber Growth: Eat more whole grains, fruits, and vegetables to gradually increase your dietary fiber intake. Although fiber encourages regularity in the digestive system, it might initially be difficult for some people with gastritis.

15. Regular Meal Schedule: Follow a regular eating pattern that includes modest, frequent

meals. Skipping meals might cause overeating, which may make the symptoms of gastritis worse.

16. Keep a Food Journal: To keep track of the things that make you sick, think about keeping a food journal. You can discover and prevent certain irritants in the future with the use of this useful tool.

17. Speak with a dietitian: Consult a certified dietitian for individualized advice and meal planning designed to meet your unique requirements due to gastritis. They may assist you in designing a diet that fits your food choices and aims for symptom control. In conclusion, learning cooking techniques and ideas for a gastritis-friendly diet requires a conscientious approach to component choice and cooking processes.

You may eat delectable meals that fuel your body while promoting digestive comfort by selecting mild cooking techniques, limiting fats, and introducing calming spices and herbs. To successfully manage gastritis, keep in mind that each person may have different tolerances for certain meals and cooking techniques. As a result, it's important to pay attention to your body and make necessary modifications.

107

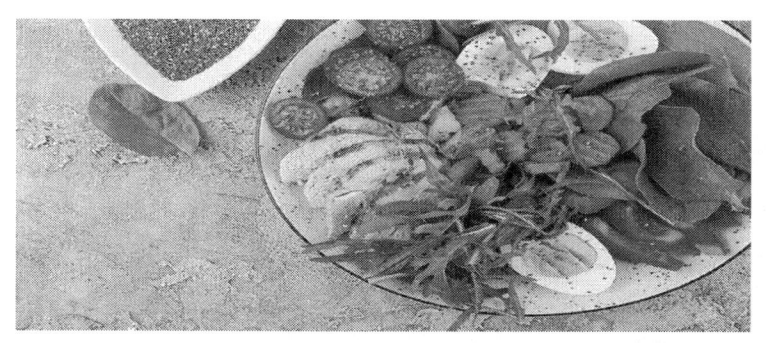

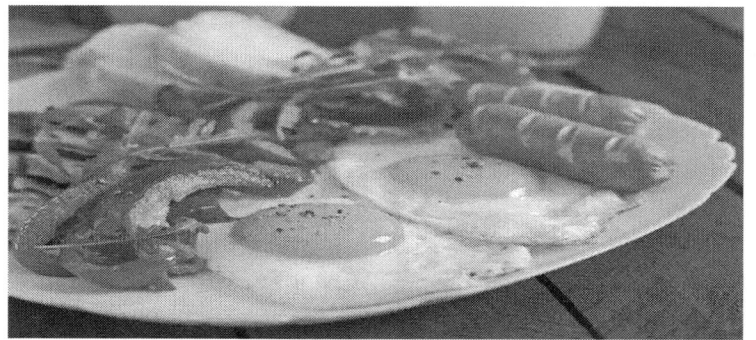

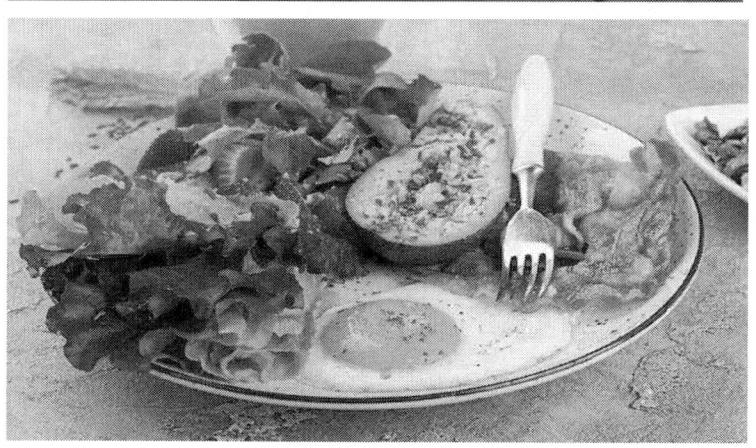

CHAPTER FOUR

Recipes for a Gastritis-Friendly Breakfast

Bananas and honey-baked oatmeal

Ingredients
1/2 cup rolled oats and
1 cup lactose-free milk or water.
1 ripe banana, sliced
Optional honey, one tablespoon;
Optional powdered flax seeds, a little quantity;

Instructions
1. In a saucepan, combine the rolled oats and the lactose-free milk or water.

2. Over low to medium heat, stir often for approximately 5-7 minutes, or until the oats are tender and the mixture thickens.

3. Remove it from the flames and give it a moment to cool.

4. If desired, top with a sliced banana and a little honey.

5. To add extra fiber and nutrients to the meal, you may alternatively add ground flaxseeds.

Eggs in a Spinach Scramble

Ingredients
2 large eggs.
1 cup finely chopped fresh spinach;
season with salt and pepper.
1 teaspoon of butter or olive oil is optional.

Instructions
1. In a bowl, beat the eggs well with a whisk.

2. Warm up a nonstick pan over low to medium heat.

3. You may, if you'd like, add some butter or olive oil to the skillet.

4. After adding it, boil the spinach for one minute, or until it wilts.

5. Pour the beaten eggs into the skillet and stir them gently while they fry.

6. Cook the eggs more until they are fully set but still moist.

7. Season the dish with salt and pepper to taste.

Greek yogurt parfait

Ingredients
1 cup plain Greek yogurt,
A small quantity of chopped nuts (such as almonds or walnuts)
For decoration half a cup of fresh berries, such as strawberries, blueberries, and raspberries.

Instructions
1. Divide the Greek yogurt in half and serve it in glasses or dishes.

2. Add a layer of fresh berries on top of the yogurt.

3. If you'd like to add a touch of sweetness, sprinkle it with honey.

4. The remaining yogurt should be positioned as the fourth layer.

5. To give the garnish extra flavor and crunch, add chopped nuts.

Chicken with ginger rice congee

Ingredients
A single tiny boneless, skinless chicken breast that has been thinly sliced;
a piece of fresh ginger that is 1 inch long;
salt and pepper to taste;
2 cups of water or low-sodium chicken broth;
1/2 cup of long- or jasmine-grain rice;

Instructions
1. Give the rice a thorough rinse.

2. Fill a pot with the rice, water, or chicken stock.

3. Bring to a boil, reduce the heat to a simmer, and cook for 30 minutes or more, stirring occasionally, or until the rice is cooked through and the mixture has thickened.

4. Add the thinly sliced chicken and grated ginger to the saucepan.

5. Continue cooking for an additional 10 to 15 minutes, or until the chicken is cooked all the way through.

6. Season with salt and pepper to taste.

7. Before serving, garnish with finely chopped green onions.

Berries Smoothie Bowl

Ingredients

1 cup plain Greek yogurt,
1/2 cup of mixed berries (strawberries, blueberries, and raspberries), plus
1 tablespoon of optional honey
1/4 cup granola (choose one with minimal sugar and no nuts).

Ingredients
1. In a dish, start with Greek yogurt as the base.

2. Add a layer of mixed berries on top of the yogurt.

3. Drizzle honey over it to give it a little more sweetness.

4. To give the berries more texture and crunch, add granola.

Banana and almond butter toast

Ingredients
1 slice of toasted whole-grain bread and
1 slice of ripe banana

one spoonful of sugar and almond butter
An optional garnish of cinnamon powder

Ingredients
1. Lightly brown the whole-grain bread while toasting.

2. Spread an equal amount of almond butter over the bread.

3. Place the banana slices on top.

4. If you want to add extra flavor, you may top it with a little ground cinnamon.

Vegetables with tofu scrambled

Ingredients
1/2 cup crumbled firm tofu and
1/4 cup chopped red, green, or yellow bell peppers
1/4 cup of sliced zucchini and tomatoes;
1/4 teaspoon of powdered turmeric;
salt and pepper to taste;

one tablespoon of olive oil

Instructions

1. Heat a nonstick skillet over low to medium heat:

2. You may optionally add some olive oil to 1.

3. Include the vegetables that have been diced and sauté them for a few minutes until they soften.

4. Add the powdered turmeric and tofu that have been crushed.

5. Continue to simmer, stirring gently, until the veggies are soft and the tofu is well cooked.

6. Season with salt and pepper to taste.

Rice Cakes with Avocado and Smoked Salmon

Ingredients

Two rice cakes.
A sliced, half-ripe avocado Smoked salmon,
2 oz. Optional garnish of fresh dill;
Serving lemon wedges, if desired

Instructions

1. Arrange the rice cakes on a dish.

2. Add sliced avocado to the top of each rice cake.

3. On top of the avocado, spread a layer of smoked salmon.

4. If preferred, garnish with fresh dill.

5. Add lemon wedges to the dish for flavor.

Berry-topped Chia Pudding

Ingredients
Chia seeds, 3 teaspoons
1 cup lactose-free milk or almond milk
One tablespoon of optional honey;

half a cup of mixed berries (strawberries, blueberries, and raspberries); and
sliced almonds as a garnish, if desired.

Instructions
1. Chia seeds and lactose-free milk should be combined in a dish. Stir well.

2. Put the mixture in the fridge for at least two hours or overnight to allow it to thicken.

3. Just before serving, mix the chia pudding to ensure a consistent consistency.

4. Top with mixed berries and, if desired, a little honey for sweetness.

5. To add extra texture, serve with sliced almonds.

Smoothie with bananas and peanut butter

Ingredients
one ripe banana

2 tablespoons pure, unrefined sugar peanut butter

1 cup lactose-free milk or almond milk

1/2 cup plain Greek yogurt

Optional spoonful of honey; a few ice cubes

Instructions

1. Put all of the ingredients in a blender.

2. Blend until creamy and smooth.

3. If you'd like it to be sweeter, taste it and add honey.

4. Include the ice cubes and mix one more, just until blended.

5. Pour your peanut butter and banana smoothie into a glass and enjoy.

Baked apple oatmeal

Ingredients

1 cup lactose-free milk or almond milk and
1/2 cup rolled oats
1 medium apple, chopped after being peeled, cored, and cooled;
1 tablespoon honey;
1/4 teaspoon cinnamon, ground
A little nutmeg
Optional garnish of chopped walnuts

Instructions

1. Set the oven's temperature to 350°F (175°C).

2. Combine rolled oats, lactose-free milk, chopped apples, honey (if preferred), ground cinnamon, and nutmeg in an ovenproof dish.

3. Combine thoroughly, then bake for 30-35 minutes, or until the apples and oats are soft.

4. Take the dish out of the oven, top with chopped walnuts if you want, and serve it hot.

Omelet with spinach and feta

Ingredients
Two big eggs.
1/4 cup chopped fresh spinach;
2 tablespoons feta cheese
Salt and pepper to taste;
cooking oil or cooking spray (optional)

Instructions
1. Beat the eggs in a bowl until well mixed.

2. Heat a nonstick pan on low to medium heat. Use a little cooking spray or olive oil if required.

3. Add the scrambled eggs to the skillet.

4. Cover one side of the omelet equally with the crumbled feta cheese and chopped spinach.

5. Permit the eggs to cook until almost set.

6. Gently fold the remaining omelet in half over the contents.

7. Cook for another few minutes, or until completely set.

8. To taste, add salt and pepper to the dish.

Quinoa Breakfast Bowl

Ingredients
1/4 cup sliced fresh strawberries,
1/4 cup sliced bananas, and
1/2 cup cooked quinoa
One tablespoon of optional honey
A garnish of finely chopped almonds (optional)

Instructions
1. Put the cooked quinoa in a bowl.

2. Add bananas and strawberry slices on top.

3. Add a drizzle of honey for extra sweetness.

4. Add chopped almonds to the garnish for taste and texture.

Cottage cheese with pineapple

Ingredients
1/2 cup low-fat cottage cheese
1/2 cup pineapple pieces in juice, not syrup, from a can
optional sprinkle of honey

Instructions
1. Put the cottage cheese in a basin.

2. Sprinkle pineapple pieces on top.

3. For an optional touch of sweetness, sprinkle honey over the dish.

4. Gently stir, then eat your breakfast that is high in protein.

Blueberry pancakes (gluten-free)

Ingredients
1/2 cup pancake mix without gluten
A quarter cup of fresh blueberries

1/4 cup almond milk or lactose-free milk
1 egg;
a half teaspoon of vanilla extract
Optional: A little quantity of pan safe frying spray or oil

Instructions
1. Combine the pancake mix, egg, lactose-free milk, and vanilla essence in a bowl.

2. Carefully incorporate fresh blueberries.

3. Put a nonstick skillet on the stovetop at medium heat. If necessary, use cooking spray or a tiny bit of oil.

4. Spoon pancake batter onto the griddle in small amounts.

5. Once bubbles appear on the surface, turn the food over and continue cooking until both sides are golden brown.

6. If tolerated, add some honey or maple syrup on top before serving.

Rice pudding with cinnamon

Ingredients
1 cup lactose-free milk or almond milk and
1/2 cup cooked white rice
One tablespoon of optional honey;
1/4 teaspoon cinnamon powder
a dash of nutmeg
Dried cranberries or raisins as a garnish (optional)

Instructions
1. Combine cooked rice, lactose-free milk, honey (if preferred), cinnamon powder, and nutmeg in a pot.

2. Cook the mixture over low heat for 15-20 minutes, stirring regularly, until it thickens.

3. Take it off the fire and let it cool.

4. If preferred, garnish with raisins or dried cranberries.

5. For a hearty breakfast alternative, serve warm.

Peanut Butter and Banana Toast

Ingredients
1 piece of toasted whole-grain bread;
1 tablespoon sugar-free natural peanut butter
a ripe banana, cut in half.
optional sprinkle of honey

Instructions
1. Toasted whole-grain bread should have a light brown color.

2. Cover the bread with an equal layer of peanut butter.

3. Position the slices of banana on top.

4. You may sprinkle a little honey on top if you'd like some more sweetness.

Rice cake topped with cottage cheese and berries

Components
1 rice cake;
one-fourth cup of low-fat cottage cheese;
a quarter cup of mixed berries, such as blueberries and raspberries
Optional garnish of ground cinnamon

Steps
1. Arrange the rice cake on a plate.

2. Cover the rice cake with a thin layer of low-fat cottage cheese.

3. Add mixed berries on top.

4. You can add a small amount of ground cinnamon for flavor.

Scrambled eggs with tomatoes and herbs

Ingredients

two big eggs.

Fresh basil or parsley, chopped (for garnish)

1/2 cup diced tomatoes;

taste-tested amounts of salt and pepper

Cooking spray or a dab of olive oil (optional)

Instructions

1. Beat the eggs in a bowl until well mixed.

2. Heat a nonstick pan on low to medium heat. If necessary, apply a little olive oil or cooking spray.

3. Add the scrambled eggs to the skillet.

4. Include the diced tomatoes and add salt and pepper to taste.

5. Cook while gently stirring until the eggs are completely set.

6. To add flavor, garnish with finely chopped fresh basil or parsley.

Banana Almond Smoothie

Ingredients
1 banana that is ripe
1 cup almond milk or lactose-free milk
1 tablespoon of sugar free almond butter
One-fourth of a teaspoon of vanilla extract
Several ice cubes

Instructions
1. Put all of the ingredients in a blender.

2. Blend until creamy and smooth.

3. Include ice cubes and blend once more to fully incorporate.

4. Pour the smoothie with the banana and almonds into a glass and savor.

Creamy Polenta with Berries

Ingredients

1/2 cup of cornmeal (polenta).

2 cups of almond milk or lactose-free milk

1 tablespoon of honey (optional)

1/2 cup of mixed berries, such as strawberries and blueberries

Instructions

1. Heat lactose-free milk to a simmer in a saucepan.

2. Cook over low heat, constantly stirring, until it thickens (typically takes 10–15 minutes). Slowly mix in the polenta.

3. Take it off the fire and let it cool.

4. Add mixed berries over top and, if you like, sprinkle with honey.

Chia Seed Breakfast Pudding

Ingredients

3 tablespoons chia seeds;

1 cup lactose-free milk or almond milk

1/2 teaspoon vanilla extract;
1 tablespoon honey (optional)
Sliced strawberries for garnish (optional)

Instructions
1. In a dish, blend chia seeds, lactose-free milk, vanilla essence, and honey (if preferred).

2. To enable the mixture to thicken, place it in the refrigerator for at least two hours or overnight.

3. To achieve a uniform consistency, stir the chia pudding just before serving.

4. Top with cut strawberries for additional freshness.

Mashed Banana and Rice Cakes

Ingredients
Two rice cakes.
1 ripe banana, mashed
A sprinkle of powdered cinnamon (optional) and

a drizzle of honey (optional)

Instructions

1. Place the rice cakes on a platter.

2. Spread the mashed banana equally over the rice cakes.

3. Optionally, sprinkle with ground cinnamon for added taste.

4. Drizzle with honey if desired for sweetness.

Creamy Coconut Rice Pudding

Ingredients

1/2 cup cooked white rice;
1/2 cup coconut milk (lactose-free)
1 tablespoon honey (optional) and
a little amount of garnished coconut shreds

Instructions

1. Combine the cooked rice and coconut milk in a saucepan.

2. Cook the mixture over low heat for 15-20 minutes, stirring regularly, until it thickens.

3. Take it off the fire and let it cool.

4. You may add honey for sweetness if you want.

5. Add a dash of coconut shavings as a garnish.

Spinach and Mushroom Scramble

Ingredients
two big eggs.
1/4 cup sliced mushrooms
1/2 cup chopped fresh spinach;
taste-tested amounts of salt and pepper;
cooking spray or a dab of olive oil (optional)

Instructions
1. Beat the eggs in a bowl until well mixed.

2. Heat a nonstick pan on low to medium heat. If necessary, use olive oil or cooking spray.

3. Include the mushroom slices and sauté them until they start to soften.

4. Add the spinach and continue to cook until the spinach wilts.

5. Scramble the eggs and add them to the skillet.

6. Cook the eggs while gently stirring until they are completely set.

7. To taste, add salt and pepper to the dish.

Rice Cake with Peanut Butter and Jelly

Ingredients
two rice cakes.
2 tablespoons of natural, sugar-free peanut butter
2 teaspoons of fruit preserves without added sugar (such as raspberry or strawberry).

Procedures

1. Arrange the rice cakes on a platter.

2. Cover one rice cake with a uniform layer of peanut butter.

3. Cover the second rice cake with fruit preserves.

4. To make a sandwich out of peanut butter and jelly, press the two rice cakes together.

Greek yogurt with baked sweet potatoes

Ingredients
1/2 cup plain Greek yogurt and
1 small sweet potato.
A sprinkling of powdered cinnamon (optional) and
A drizzle of honey

Instructions

1. Prick the sweet potato with a fork and bake it for 45–60 minutes, or until tender, at 375°F (190°C).

2. Cut the sweet potato in half, then use a fork to fluff the flesh.

3. Add some plain Greek yogurt on top.

4. To enhance flavor, you may pour honey over the dish and add ground cinnamon.

Nutty Quinoa Porridge

Ingredients
1/4 cup chopped mixed nuts (such as almonds and walnuts) and
1/2 cup cooked quinoa
1/4 cup of thinly sliced fresh fruit (apple, pear, etc.)
optional sprinkle of honey

Instructions
1. In a bowl, add the cooked quinoa.

2. Add fresh fruit slices and chopped mixed nuts on top.

3. You may sprinkle honey on top if you'd like more sweetness.

4. Gently stir, then eat your filling quinoa porridge.

Chia and Berry Breakfast Bowl Left Over

Ingredients
Three tablespoons of chia seeds
1 cup almond milk or lactose-free milk
1/2 cup of mixed berries (such as strawberries and blueberries).
One tablespoon of optional honey
Optional garnish: sliced almonds

Instructions
1. Combine chia seeds and lactose-free milk in a dish. Stir well.

2. To enable the mixture to thicken, place it in the refrigerator for at least 4 hours or overnight.

3. To achieve a uniform consistency, stir the chia pudding just before serving.

4. Add mixed berries over top and, if you like, sprinkle with honey.

5. Add sliced almonds as a garnish for more texture.

Cinnamon Apple Porridge

Ingredients
1 cup lactose-free milk or almond milk and
1/2 cup rolled oats.
1 small apple, diced after being peeled, cored, and drained.
Optional sprinkle of honey

Instructions
1. Combine the rolled oats, apple dice, cinnamon, and lactose-free milk in a saucepan.

2. Cook, stirring periodically, over low heat for 5-7 minutes, or until the oats are cooked and the mixture thickens.

3. Take it off the fire and let it cool.

4. You may sprinkle honey on top if you'd like more sweetness.

5. Delight in your cozy cinnamon apple porridge.

Yogurt and Fruit Parfait

Ingredients
1 cup Greek yogurt, plain
1 tablespoon of honey (optional)
1/2 cup of fresh mixed berries (such as blueberries and raspberries)
A small handful of low-sugar granola for garnish

Instructions

1.Layer half of the plain Greek yogurt in a glass or dish.

2. Top the yogurt with a layer of mixed berries.

3. If desired, drizzle with honey.

4. The fourth layer should be the leftover yogurt.

5. To add crunch and taste, garnish with granola.

Warm banana cereal

Ingredients
1 cup almond milk or lactose-free milk
1/2 cup rice cereal (choose one without sugar added).
Sliced banana, 1 ripe banana, and
optional ground cinnamon

Instructions
1. Heat lactose-free milk in a saucepan over low to medium heat.

2. Add the rice cereal and simmer, stirring constantly, for about 5-7 minutes, or until it thickens.

3. Take it off the fire and let it cool.

4. Add sliced banana on top, and you may choose to add some ground cinnamon for taste.

Creamy Pumpkin Oatmeal

Ingredients
1 cup lactose-free milk or almond milk and
1/2 cup rolled oats.
1/4 cup of unsweetened canned pumpkin puree
A mixture of cinnamon, nutmeg, and cloves, or
1/2 teaspoon pumpkin pie spice
optional sprinkle of maple syrup

Instructions
1. Combine pumpkin puree, lactose-free milk, rolled oats, and pumpkin pie spice in a saucepan.

2. Cook for about 5-7 minutes, or until the oats are soft and the mixture thickens, over low to medium heat, stirring regularly.

3. Take it off the fire and let it cool.

4. You may spray maple syrup on top if you'd like more sweetness.

5. Enjoy your creamy porridge with pumpkin.

Poached eggs with spinach and tomato

Ingredients
Two big eggs.
1/2 cup chopped tomatoes;
1 cup fresh spinach leaves
Taste-tested amounts of salt and pepper
Cooking spray or a dab of olive oil (optional)

Instructions
1. Heat the water in a pan until it is simmering.

2. If necessary, apply cooking spray or a tiny bit of olive oil.

3. Gently break the eggs into the boiling water, then poach them for 3 to 4 minutes, or until the whites are set but the yolks are still a little liquid.

4. Using a slotted spoon, remove the poached eggs from the water.

5. Sauté the diced tomatoes and fresh spinach in the same pan until the spinach wilts.

6. Top the spinach and tomato mixture with the poached eggs.

7. To taste, add salt and pepper to the dish. With a variety of tastes and ingredients, these extra breakfast ideas will keep your morning meals flavorful and gastritis-friendly.

Almond Butter and Banana Smoothie Bowl

Ingredients

1 banana that is ripe
2 tablespoons of sugar-free, natural almond butter
1/2 cup almond milk or lactose-free milk
A few sliced almonds as a garnish (optional)
Fresh banana slices as a topping, if desired.

Instructions
1. Blend the ripe banana, almond butter, and lactose-free milk in a blender.

2. Blend until creamy and smooth.

3. Place a bowl with the smoothie inside.

4. To add texture and taste, sprinkle some sliced almonds and fresh banana slices over top.

Savory Quinoa Breakfast Bowl

Ingredients
1/4 cup sautéed spinach and mushrooms, and
1/2 cup cooked quinoa.
1 poached or soft-boiled egg;

A dash of salt and pepper
Finely chopped fresh herbs (parsley, chives, etc.) for garnish

Instructions
1. In a bowl, add the cooked quinoa.

2. Add mushrooms and spinach that have been sautéed.

3. Include a soft-boiled or poached egg.

4. Add a little salt and pepper for seasoning.

5. To add more taste, garnish with finely chopped fresh herbs.

Chia pudding with mango and coconut

Ingredients
Three tablespoons of chia seeds
1 cup lactose-free coconut milk
One-half of a diced, juicy mango;
A sprinkle of honey (optional)

Instructions

1. Combine coconut milk and chia seeds in a dish. Stir well.

2. To enable the mixture to thicken, place it in the refrigerator for at least two hours or overnight.

3. To achieve a uniform consistency, stir the chia pudding just before serving.

4. Add diced ripe mango over top and, if you like, sprinkle with honey.

Scrambled tofu breakfast burrito

Ingredients
1/4 cup chopped red, green, or yellow bell peppers and
1/2 cup crumbled firm tofu.
1/4 cup tomatoes, diced
1/4 teaspoon of powdered turmeric;
To taste-sized salt and pepper

1 whole-wheat tortilla

Instructions

1. In a pan, cook chopped tomatoes and bell peppers until they are soft.

2. Include turmeric powder and crushed firm tofu.

3. Heat the tofu thoroughly while gently stirring.

4. To taste, add salt and pepper to the dish.

5. Get the whole-wheat tortilla warm.

6. To make a breakfast burrito, spread the tofu scramble on the tortilla and fold it up.

Peach and Rice Cereal Bowl

Ingredients:
1 cup of rice cereal (choose one without sugar added).
1/8 of a sliced ripe peach;

one tablespoon of optional honey;
an optional garnish of ground cinnamon

Instructions:
1. Put the rice cereal in a bowl.

2. Add sliced, juicy peaches on top.

3. To make it sweeter, drizzle with honey.

4. You may add ground cinnamon as an optional garnish for more taste.

Cottage cheese and pineapple parfait

Ingredients
1/2 cup low-fat cottage cheese
1/2 cup sliced pineapple in juice (not syrup) from a can
optional sprinkle of honey

Instructions:
1. Put the low-fat cottage cheese in a bowl.

2. Top with diced pineapple.

3. For an optional touch of sweetness, sprinkle honey over the dish.

4. Gently combine, then enjoy your protein-packed parfait.

Oatmeal with blueberries and almonds

Ingredients
1 cup lactose-free milk or almond milk and 1/2 cup rolled oats.
A quarter cup of fresh blueberries
1 tablespoon of sugar free almond butter
An optional sprinkling of ground flaxseeds

Instructions
1. Combine lactose-free milk and rolled oats in a saucepan.

2. Cook for about 5-7 minutes, or until the oats are soft and the mixture thickens, over low to medium heat, stirring regularly.

3. Take it off the fire and let it cool.

4. Add some almond butter and fresh blueberries on top.

5. You may optionally add ground flaxseeds to the dish for more nutrients and fiber.

Strawberry Banana Smoothie Bowl

Ingredients
1 banana that is ripe;
1/2 cup of fresh strawberries
1/2 cup yogurt without lactose;
a small handful of low-sugar granola for garnish

Instructions
1. Blend the ripe banana, fresh strawberries, and lactose-free yogurt together in a blender.

2. Blend until creamy and smooth.

3. Place a bowl with the smoothie inside.

4. To add crunch and texture, sprinkle some granola over top.

Breakfast Wrap with Veggies and Cheese

Ingredients
2 scrambled eggs and
1 whole-grain tortilla
1/4 cup sautéed onions and bell peppers
1/4 cup low-fat cheese that has been chopped up
A dash of salt and pepper

Instructions
1. Get the whole-wheat tortilla warm.

2. Place scrambled eggs, sautéed bell peppers, onions, and low-fat cheese within the tortilla.

3. Add a little salt and pepper for seasoning.

4. To make a breakfast wrap, roll the tortilla up.

Rice Cakes with Cinnamon and Raisins

Ingredients
two rice cakes.
Two tablespoons of low-fat cream cheese
A dash of cinnamon powder
A few raisins for the garnish

Steps
1: Arrange the rice cakes on a platter.

2. Evenly cover the rice cakes with low-fat cream cheese.

3. Add ground cinnamon to the surface.

4. Add raisins as a garnish for extra sweetness.

Pumpkin Spice Smoothie

Ingredients
1/2 cup canned, unsweetened pumpkin puree;
a half-ripe banana
1 cup almond milk or lactose-free milk
A mixture of cinnamon, nutmeg, and cloves, or

1/4 teaspoon pumpkin pie spice;
an optional sprinkle of honey

Instructions

1. Blend canned pumpkin puree, a ripe banana, lactose-free milk, and pumpkin pie spice together in a blender.

2. Blend until well integrated and smooth.

3. You may sprinkle honey on top if you'd like more sweetness.

Veggie and Cheese Omelette

Ingredients
Two big eggs.
1/4 cup chopped tomatoes
1/4 cup diced bell peppers, either red, green, or yellow
1/4 cup low-fat cheese, shred
Taste-tested amounts of salt and pepper
Cooking spray or a dab of olive oil (optional)

Instructions

1. Beat the eggs in a bowl until well mixed.

2. Heat a nonstick pan on low to medium heat. If necessary, use a little olive oil or frying spray.

3. Add the scrambled eggs to the skillet.

4. Cover one side of the omelet equally with chopped bell peppers, diced tomatoes, and low-fat cheese.

5. Permit the eggs to cook until almost set.

6. Gently fold the remaining omelet in half over the contents.

7. Cook for another few minutes, or until completely set.

8. To taste, add salt and pepper to the dish.

Mixed Berry Chia Pudding

Ingredients

Three tablespoons of chia seeds
1 cup almond milk or lactose-free milk
1/2 cup mixed berries (e.g., blueberries, raspberries, strawberries) and
1 tablespoon honey (optional)
Optional garnish: sliced almonds

Instructions

1. Combine chia seeds and lactose-free milk in a dish. Stir well.

2. To enable the mixture to thicken, place it in the refrigerator for at least two hours or overnight.

3. To achieve a uniform consistency, stir the chia pudding just before serving.

4. Add mixed berries over top and, if you like, sprinkle with honey.

5. Add sliced almonds as a garnish for more texture.

Avocado and egg toast

Ingredients
1 piece of toasted whole-grain bread;
1/2 mashed, ripe avocado
1 soft-boiled or poached egg;
A dash of salt and pepper
Optional garnish:
Cherry tomatoes, sliced

Instructions
1. Toasted whole-grain bread should have a light brown color.

2. Cover the bread with an equal layer of mashed avocado.

3. Add a soft-boiled or poached egg on top.

4. Add a little salt and pepper for seasoning.

5. If preferred, garnish with thinly sliced cherry tomatoes.

Veggie Breakfast Bowl

Ingredients:
1/4 cup sautéed spinach and mushrooms and
1/2 cup cooked quinoa.
1 scrambled egg,
Optionally drizzled with olive oil,
Salt, and pepper

Instructions:
1. In a bowl, add the cooked quinoa.

2. Add mushrooms and spinach that have been sautéed.

3. Include a fried egg.

4. Add a little salt and pepper for seasoning.

5. You might sprinkle a little olive oil on top for taste.

Apple Cinnamon Rice Cakes

Ingredients

two rice cakes.
2 tablespoons of sugar free almond butter
A thinly cut half of an apple
A dash of cinnamon powder
optional sprinkle of honey

Steps

1: Arrange the rice cakes on a platter.

2. Cover the rice cakes with a uniform layer of almond butter.

3. Scatter apple slices thinly over the top.

4. Add ground cinnamon for additional taste.

5. You may sprinkle honey on top if you'd like more sweetness.

For a variety of tastes and ingredients to complement your gastritis-friendly morning meals, try these extra breakfast ideas. Enjoy your healthy breakfasts after customizing them to suit your tastes and dietary requirements!

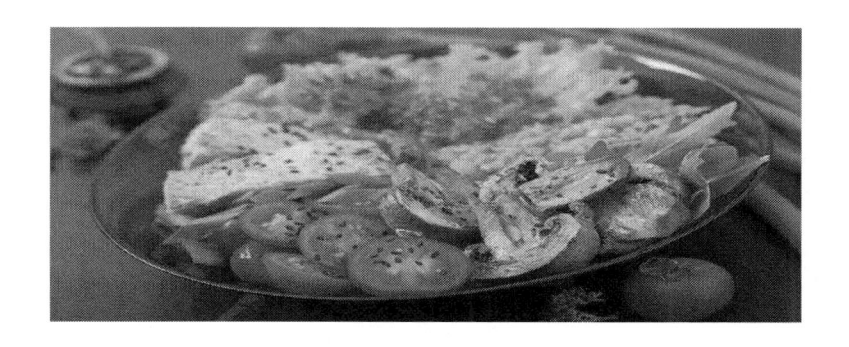

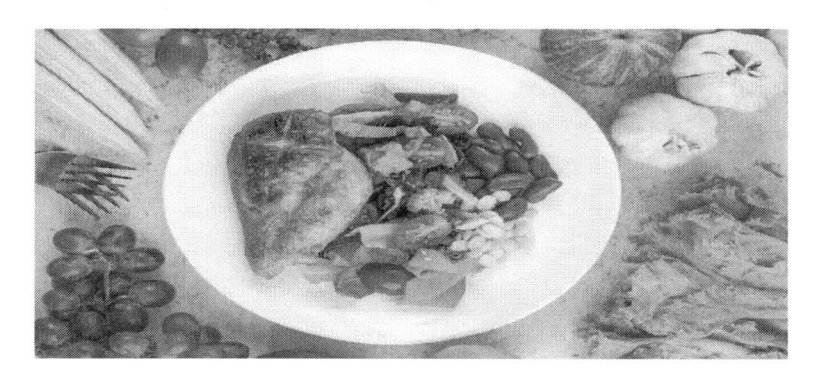

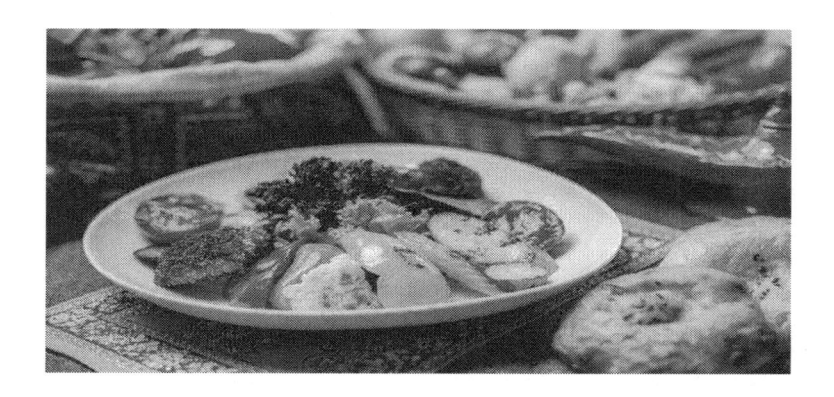

CHAPTER FIVE

Recipes for a Gastritis-Friendly Lunch

Quinoa and Grilled Chicken Bowl

Ingredient
One boneless, skinless chicken breast,
half a cup of quinoa,
one cup of low-sodium chicken broth,
one cup of steamed spinach, and
half a cup of cooked, softened carrots.
Cooking with olive oil,
salt, and pepper

Instructions
1. Sprinkle a little salt and pepper on the chicken breast.

2. Set a grill or a grill pan on the stovetop to medium-high heat. Small amounts of olive oil should be brushed onto the grill.

3. Grill the chicken breast until thoroughly done, approximately 5-7 minutes per side.

4. Drain the quinoa after giving it a quick rinse under cold water while the chicken cooks.

5. Bring the low-sodium chicken stock to a boil in a different pot.

6. After adding the quinoa to the simmering soup, turn the heat down to low, cover the pot, and let the quinoa cook for 15 minutes, or until it is cooked and the liquid has been absorbed.

7. Put the cooked quinoa, steamed spinach, and cooked carrots in a bowl. Mix slowly.

8. Lay the sliced grilled chicken breast on top of the quinoa and veggie combination.

9. If you'd like more taste, drizzle with a little olive oil.

10. Offer your quinoa and grilled chicken dish as a filling and gastritis-friendly lunch choice.

Salmon baked in the oven with mashed sweet potatoes

Ingredients
One big sweet potato,
one salmon filet, and
one tablespoon of olive oil (to taste);
salt and pepper

Instructions
1. Set the oven's temperature to 375°F (190°C).

2. Rub a little salt and pepper on the salmon filet and drizzle some olive oil over it.

3. Arrange the salmon on a parchment-lined baking sheet.

4. Bake for 15-20 minutes in a preheated oven, or until the salmon flakes easily with a fork.

5. Peel and julienne the sweet potato while the fish is baking.

6. Cook the sweet potato for a few minutes to make it soft (around 10–15).

7. After draining, mash the sweet potato with a fork or potato masher.

8. Add a little olive oil, salt, and pepper to taste as you season the mashed sweet potato.

9. For a delightful and comforting meal, serve the cooked salmon with the mashed sweet potatoes.

Wrap with turkey and avocado

Ingredients
One whole-wheat tortilla
4 slices of low-sodium roasted turkey breast
A sliced, half-ripe avocado
1 finely sliced tiny cucumber;

1 cup of mixed greens (such as arugula and spinach).
Optional plain Greek yogurt dressing:
salt and pepper to taste

Instructions

1. The whole-grain tortilla should be laid out flat on a tidy surface.

2. Evenly distribute the turkey pieces over the tortilla.

3. Arrange the turkey, cucumber, avocado slices, and mixed greens on a plate.

4. To taste, add a touch of salt and pepper.

5. You may sprinkle some plain Greek yogurt over the salad as a creamy dressing.

6. To make a wrap for the turkey and avocado, fold the tortilla's edges in and roll it up securely.

7. Cut the wrap in half to have a light and cooling meal that is suitable for those with gastritis.

Stir-Fry with Quinoa and Vegetables

Ingredients
1 cup low-sodium vegetable broth;
1 cup of mixed veggies (such as bell peppers, broccoli, carrots, and snap peas)
1/2 cup quinoa
1/2 cup cubed firm tofu (optional)
- Tamari or low-sodium soy sauce for taste
- 1 tablespoon cooking sesame oil

Instructions
1. Drain the quinoa after giving it a cold water rinse.

2. Bring the low-sodium vegetable broth to a boil in a saucepan.

3. After adding the quinoa to the simmering stock, turn the heat down to low, cover the pot, and let the quinoa cook for 15 minutes.

4. In a skillet over medium heat, warm the sesame oil while the quinoa is cooking.

5. Add the mixed veggies to the skillet and stir-fry with the tofu (if using) until the vegetables are soft.

6. When the quinoa has finished cooking, fluff it with a fork and add it to the skillet with the tofu and veggies.

7. For taste, drizzle with tamari or low-sodium soy sauce.

8. Combine everything and dish out the quinoa and veggie stir-fry.

Vegetable and Lentil Soup

Ingredients

4 cups of low-sodium vegetable broth,
1/2 cup dry green or brown lentils, and
1 cup of mixed veggies (such as carrots, celery, and zucchini).
1/2 cup chopped tomatoes, salt-free from a can;
half a teaspoon of dried thyme;
to taste, salt and pepper

Instructions

1. Drain the lentils after giving them a cold water rinse.

2. Combine the lentils, low-sodium vegetable broth, diced tomatoes, mixed veggies, dried thyme, salt, and pepper in a big saucepan.

3. Bring the mixture to a boil, then lower the heat to a simmer, covering the pan, and cook for 25 to 30 minutes, or until the lentils are cooked.

4. Taste your hearty lentil and vegetable soup, and add more salt and pepper if necessary.

Chicken Breast Stuffed with Spinach and Feta

Ingredients
1 cup of fresh spinach leaves;
1 boneless, skinless chicken breast
One tablespoon of low-fat, shredded feta cheese;
To-taste salt and pepper
Cooking oil made from olives

Instructions
1. Set the oven's temperature to 375°F (190°C).

2. Be cautious not to cut all the way through the chicken breast while creating a pocket in the side.

3. Sprinkle a little salt and pepper within the pocket.

4. Insert some feta cheese and new spinach leaves into the pocket.

5. In a skillet that can be used in the oven, warm a little olive oil over medium-high heat.

6. Lightly brown the chicken breast by searing it for two to three minutes on each side.

7. Place the pan in the hot oven and bake for 15-20 minutes, or until the chicken is fully done.

8. Serve your chicken breast filled with spinach and feta as a filling and gastritis-friendly meal.

Tuna and white bean salad

Ingredients
1 can (5 ounces) of drained water-packed tuna
1 cup washed and drained canned white beans (cannellini or navy beans)
1 lemon's worth of juice
1/2 cup sliced cucumber
1/4 cup diced red onion;
1/4 cup chopped fresh parsley;
optional dressing made with olive oil
To taste, salt and pepper

Instructions

1. Combine the white beans, diced cucumber, diced red onion, and fresh parsley in a dish along with the drained tuna.

2. Sprinkle the mixture with lemon juice.

3. To enhance flavor, you may sprinkle a little bit of olive oil on top.

4. To taste, add salt and pepper to the dish.

5. Combine everything and dish out your light tuna and white bean salad.

Quinoa with Roasted Vegetable Salad

Ingredients
2 cups of mixed roasted veggies (such as bell peppers, zucchini, and cherry tomatoes)
1/2 cup of quinoa
1 cup of low-sodium vegetable broth
1/4 cup goat cheese crumbles (optional)

low-sodium balsamic vinaigrette dressing, if desired

To taste, salt and pepper

Instructions

1. Drain the quinoa after giving it a cold water rinse.

2. Bring the low-sodium vegetable broth to a boil in a saucepan.

3. After adding the quinoa to the simmering stock, turn the heat down to low, cover the pot, and let the quinoa cook for 15 minutes.

4. Roast the mixed veggies in the oven at 400°F (200°C) for 20 to 25 minutes, or until they are soft, while the quinoa cooks.

5. Combine the quinoa and veggies in a bowl after they are both done.

6. Goat cheese crumbles are an optional addition to enhance richness.

7. For taste, drizzle with balsamic vinaigrette dressing.

8. To taste, add salt and pepper to the dish.

9. Offer your quinoa and roasted veggie salad as a filling and healthy lunch option.

Omelet with eggs and spinach

Ingredients
2 eggs, big
One cup of new spinach leaves
1/4 cup chopped bell peppers, your choice of color;
1/4 cup chopped tomatoes, salt-free from a can;
cooking with olive oil;
salt and pepper to taste

Instructions
1. Beat the eggs in a bowl until well mixed.

2. In case more olive oil is required, preheat a nonstick skillet over medium-low heat.

3. Add the scrambled eggs to the skillet.

4. Add the chopped tomatoes, bell peppers, and fresh spinach leaves to one side of the omelet as the eggs begin to set.

5. To taste, add a touch of salt and pepper.

6. Gently fold the remaining omelet in half over the contents.

7. Cook the dish for a few more minutes until it is completely set.

8. Transfer the omelet to a tray and serve the egg and spinach dish as a wholesome and light meal.

A bowl of brown rice and salmon

Ingredients
1 salmon filet,

1 cup brown rice,
1 cup broccoli that has been steam-cooked, and 1/2 cup shredded carrots.
Optional low-sodium soy sauce for drizzling
- Optional garnish: sesame seeds;
salt and pepper to taste

Instructions

1. Add a dash of salt and pepper to the salmon filet.

2. Put a nonstick skillet on the stovetop at medium-high heat.

3. Cook the salmon for 4 to 5 minutes on each side, depending on how done you want it.

4. Combine the steamed broccoli, shredded carrots, and brown rice in a bowl.

5. To add more flavor, drizzle with low-sodium soy sauce.

6. Top the rice and veggies with the cooked salmon.

7. If you'd like, add sesame seeds as a garnish.

8. Present your salmon and brown rice dish for a wholesome and gastritis-friendly meal.

Stir-fried turkey and vegetables

Ingredients
1 cup sliced cooked turkey breast
1 cup stirred mixture
-fry veggies (such as bell peppers, mushrooms, and snap peas)
low-sodium sauce for stir-fries
1 cup of prepared quinoa or rice
Cooking with olive oil
To taste, salt and pepper

Instructions
1. In a large skillet or wok, heat the olive oil over medium-high heat.

2. Include the mixed veggies in the stir-fry and heat until they begin to soften.

3. Include the stir-fry sauce and thinly sliced turkey breast.

4. Continue to cook for an additional 2-3 minutes to fully reheat everything.

5. Put cooked quinoa or rice on top of the stir-fry with turkey and vegetables.

6. To taste, add salt and pepper.

7. Indulge in a short and tasty meal.

A wrap with hummus and vegetables

Ingredients
One whole-wheat tortilla
1/4 cup low-fat hummus
1/2 cup of mixed raw veggies (such as baby spinach, bell peppers, and cucumbers)
1/4 cup thinly sliced black olives

To taste, salt and pepper

Instructions

1. The whole-grain tortilla should be laid out flat on a tidy surface.

2. Cover the tortilla with a uniform coating of hummus.

3. Place the sliced black olives and the mixed raw veggies on top.

4. To taste, add a touch of salt and pepper.

5. Fold the tortilla's edges in and wrap it up securely.

6. Cut the wrap in half, then eat the filling and wholesome hummus and vegetable wrap.

Lentil and spinach salad

Ingredients
2 cups of fresh spinach leaves;

1/2 cup of cooked green or brown lentils;
1/4 cup chopped cucumber; and
1/4 cup diced red bell pepper
- Low-sodium balsamic vinaigrette dressing, if desired;
- To taste, salt and pepper

Instructions
1. Combine the chopped red bell pepper, diced cucumber, fresh spinach leaves, and cooked lentils in a dish.

2. For taste, drizzle with balsamic vinaigrette dressing.

3. To taste, add salt and pepper to the dish.

4. Combine everything and serve the lentil and spinach salad as a filling and light meal.

Bell peppers stuffed with turkey and quinoa

Ingredients
2 bell peppers, big

1 cup cooked quinoa;
1 cup cooked lean, low-sodium ground turkey;
1/4 cup chopped tomatoes, salt-free from a can;
to taste, salt and pepper

Instructions

1. Set the oven's temperature to 375°F (190°C).

2. Cut the bell peppers' tops off and scoop out the seeds and membranes.

3. Combine cooked ground turkey, cooked quinoa, and diced tomatoes in a bowl.

4. To taste, add salt and pepper to the dish.

5. Stuff the quinoa and turkey mixture into the bell peppers.

6. Put the peppers on a baking tray after being filled.

7. Bake the peppers for 25 to 30 minutes, or until they are soft, in a preheated oven while they are covered in foil.

8. Offer your quinoa and turkey-stuffed bell peppers as a filling and healthy lunch option.

Chickpea and Cucumber Salad

Ingredients
1 can (15 ounces) of washed and drained chickpeas
1/2 diced cucumber;
1/4 cup minced fresh parsley;
1/4 cup diced red onion
1 lemon's juice
Optional dressing made with olive oil
To taste, salt and pepper

Instructions
1. Combine the chickpeas, diced red onion, diced cucumber, and chopped fresh parsley in a bowl.

2. Sprinkle the mixture with lemon juice.

3. To enhance flavor, you may sprinkle a little bit of olive oil on top.

4. To taste, add salt and pepper to the dish.

5. Combine all of the ingredients, then serve your chickpea and cucumber salad as a light and protein-rich lunch.

Salad made with roasted butternut squash and lentils

Ingredients
Cooked green or brown lentils,
1 cup–2 cups roasted butternut squash cubes with
Salt, pepper, and olive oil.
1/4 cup freshly chopped parsley;
two teaspoons of low-sodium balsamic vinegar, if you'd like.
Optional dressing made with olive oil,
salt, and pepper

Instructions

1. Combine the cooked lentils, cubes of roasted butternut squash, and fresh parsley in a bowl.

2. For taste, drizzle some olive oil and balsamic vinegar over top.

3. To taste, add salt and pepper to the food.

4. Serve your roasted butternut squash and lentil salad as a filling and healthy lunch by tossing everything together.

Avocado with Shrimp Salad

Ingredients
1 cup peeled, cooked shrimp;
a sliced, half-ripe avocado;
1 cup of mixed greens, such as arugula and baby spinach.
Halved cherry tomatoes;
lemon juice drizzled over food;
optional dressing made with olive oil

salt and pepper to taste

Instructions
1. The cooked shrimp, sliced avocado, mixed greens, and cherry tomatoes should all be combined in a dish.

2. For taste, drizzle with lemon juice and/or olive oil.

3. To taste, add salt and pepper to the food.

4. Serve your shrimp and avocado salad as a light and energizing lunch by tossing everything together.

Omelet with spinach and mushrooms

Ingredients
2 eggs, big;
one cup of new spinach leaves;
a serving of sliced mushrooms
one-fourth cup diced onion;
cooking with olive oil;

To taste; salt and pepper

Instructions

1. Beat the eggs in a bowl until they are fully mixed.

2. If necessary, heat a non-stick skillet over low heat with a tiny quantity of olive oil.

3. To the pan, add the chopped onion and the sliced mushrooms, and cook until the mushrooms are tender.

4. Over the sautéed veggies, pour the beaten eggs.

5. On top of the eggs, place the fresh spinach leaves.

6. To taste, add a touch of salt and pepper.

7. Fold the omelet in half with care.

8. Once completely set, cook for a few minutes longer.

9. Serve your spinach and mushroom omelet as a filling meal by sliding it onto a dish.

Curry with tofu and vegetables

Ingredients
- A diced 1/2 brick of firm tofu
- 1 cup of mixed veggies, such as carrots, broccoli, and bell peppers
- 1/2 cup chopped tomatoes, salt-free from a can
- A quarter cup of light coconut milk
- Low-sodium curry powder or paste, if available
- Cooking with olive oil
- To taste, salt and pepper

Instructions
1. In a pan over medium heat, warm the olive oil.

2. Add the tofu cubes and continue cooking until just browned.

3. When the mixed veggies are added, add a few more minutes of sautéing to bring out their softness.

4. Add the chopped tomatoes, light coconut milk, and curry powder or paste while adjusting the heat to your preference.

5. Simmer the veggies for 10 to 15 minutes, or until they are soft.

6. To taste, add salt and pepper to the food.

7. For a tasty and filling lunch, serve your tofu and vegetable curry over cooked brown rice or quinoa.

Grilled chicken with Greek Salad

Ingredients
a single skinless, boneless chicken breast;
one cup of mixed greens, such as romaine lettuce, cucumbers, and cherry tomatoes;

a quarter cup of crumbled low-fat feta cheese;
Pitted and sliced Kalamata olives;
A low-sodium balsamic vinaigrette dressing, if desired; and,
To taste, salt and pepper.

Instructions

1. Sprinkle a little salt and pepper on the chicken breast to season.

2. Over medium-high heat, preheat a grill or a grill pan on the stove.

3. The chicken breast should be cooked through on the grill for approximately 5-7 minutes on each side.

4. Prepare a salad with mixed greens, feta cheese crumbles, and sliced Kalamata olives while the chicken is cooking.

5. For taste, drizzle with balsamic vinaigrette dressing.

6. Sliced chicken should be added to the salad once the chicken has finished cooking.

7. To taste, add salt and pepper to the food.

8. For an energizing and protein-rich meal, combine your Greek salad with grilled chicken.

Bell Peppers Stuffed with Veggies and Quinoa

Ingredients
2 bell peppers, big;
1 serving of cooked quinoa;
1 cup of mixed veggies, such as chopped tomatoes, corn, and zucchini
To taste; salt and pepper;
Cooking with olive oil

Instructions
1. Set your oven's temperature to 375°F (190°C).

2. Remove the bell peppers' tops, then scoop out the seeds and membranes.

3. The cooked quinoa, mixed veggies, salt, and pepper should all be combined in a dish.

4. The quinoa and veggie mixture should be stuffed into the bell peppers.

5. The filled peppers should be put on a baking dish.

6. Bake the peppers in the preheated oven for 25 to 30 minutes, or until they are soft, covered with foil.

7. Serve your quinoa and vegetable-stuffed bell peppers as a filling and healthy lunch.

Lemon and Herbs in Baked Cod

Ingredients
1 filet of cod
- Slices of lemon
- Fresh herbs (such as rosemary and thyme)
- Drizzles of olive oil
- To taste, salt and pepper

Instructions

1. Set your oven's temperature to 375°F (190°C).

2. On a baking sheet covered with parchment paper, put the fish filet.

3. To taste, add salt and pepper to the food.

4. Lemon slices and fresh herbs go on top.

5. Add a little olive oil to the dish.

6. Bake for 15 to 20 minutes in a preheated oven, or until the cod flakes easily with a fork.

7. For a tasty and light lunch, serve your baked fish with lemon and herbs.

Tuna with cucumber salad

Ingredients
1 can (5 ounces) of drained water-packed tuna;
1/2 diced cucumber;

1/4 cup chopped red onion;
2 tablespoons of low-fat Greek yogurt, if you'd like.
- Dill for taste, fresh
- To taste, salt and pepper

Instructions
1. Tuna that has been drained, cucumber, red onion, and plain Greek yogurt should all be combined in a dish.

2. Add fresh dill for a flavor boost.

3. To taste, add salt and pepper to the food.

4. Serve your cucumber and tuna salad as a cooling and protein-rich lunch by tossing everything together.

Quiche with spinach and tomatoes

Ingredients
1 whole-grain pie crust, either handmade or purchased.

Two cups of new spinach leaves;
1 cup diced tomatoes;
4 big eggs; and
half a cup of low-fat milk, if you'd like.
1/4 cup of low-sodium Parmesan cheese, if desired.
- To taste, salt and pepper

Instructions

1. Set your oven's temperature to 375°F (190°C).

2. On a pie plate, put the whole-grain pie dough.

3. The chopped tomatoes and fresh spinach leaves should be combined in a basin.

4. Whisk the eggs, milk, Parmesan cheese, salt, and pepper in a separate bowl.

5. On top of the spinach and tomatoes, pour the egg mixture.

6. Bake the pie dish for 25 to 30 minutes, or until the quiche is set and gently browned. Carefully put the pie dish in the preheated oven.

7. Before slicing and serving your spinach and tomato quiche as a filling meal, give it a moment to cool somewhat.

Stir-fry with vegetables and chickpeas

Ingredients
1 can (15 ounces) of washed and drained chickpeas;
2 cups of a variety of stir-fried veggies, such as broccoli, bell peppers, and snap peas;
a low-sodium sauce for stir-fries;
1 cup cooked quinoa or brown rice;
Cooking with olive oil; and,
To taste, salt and pepper

Instructions
1. In a large skillet or wok, heat the olive oil over medium-high heat.

2. Stir-fry the various stir-fry veggies after adding them until they begin to soften.

3. Stir-fry sauce and chickpeas should be added.

4. Cook for a further 2 to 3 minutes, or until everything is well heated.

5. Over cooked brown rice or quinoa, top the stir-fry with vegetables and chickpeas.

6. To taste, add salt and pepper to the food.

7. Enjoy a tasty meal that is fast.

Wrap with turkey and cranberries

Ingredients
One whole-wheat tortilla;
4 slices of low-sodium roasted turkey breast;
2 tablespoons of unsweetened cranberry sauce, if you'd like.
A quarter cup of young spinach leaves;
To taste; salt and pepper.

Instructions

1. The whole-grain tortilla should be placed level on a tidy surface.

2. Spread out the tortilla with the roasted turkey pieces equally.

3. Overlay the turkey with the cranberry sauce.

4. On top, add the young spinach leaves.

5. To taste, add a touch of salt and pepper.

6. The tortilla's sides should be folded in and rolled up securely.

7. Enjoy a festive and delectable turkey and cranberry wrap by slicing it in half.

Stir-Fry with Veggies and Tofu

Ingredients
- A diced 1/2 brick of firm tofu;

2 cups of a variety of stir-fried veggies, such as broccoli, bell peppers, and carrots;
low-sodium sauce for stir-fries;
1 serving of cooked quinoa or brown rice;
cooking with olive oil
Salt and pepper to taste

Instructions

1. In a large skillet or wok, heat the olive oil over medium-high heat.

2. Stir-fry the various stir-fry veggies after adding them until they begin to soften.

3. Stir-fry sauce and diced tofu should be added.

4. Cook for a further 2 to 3 minutes until well cooked.

5. Overcooked quinoa or brown rice, plate the stir-fry with the vegetables and tofu.

6. To taste, add salt and pepper to the food.

7. Savor a tasty, high-protein meal.

Chicken Grilled with Caprese Salad

Ingredients
a single skinless, boneless chicken breast;
1 cup halved cherry tomatoes;
a half cup of cubed fresh mozzarella cheese;
fresh leaves of basil;
low-sodium balsamic vinaigrette dressing, if desired;
grilling with olive oil.
- To taste, salt and pepper

Instructions
1. Sprinkle a little salt and pepper on the chicken breast to season.

2. Over medium-high heat, preheat a grill or a grill pan on the stove.

3. The chicken breast should be cooked through on the grill for approximately 5-7 minutes on each side.

4. Prepare a salad with cherry tomatoes, fresh mozzarella cheese, and fresh basil leaves while the chicken is cooking.

5. For taste, drizzle with balsamic vinaigrette dressing.

6. Sliced chicken should be added to the salad once the chicken has finished cooking.

7. To taste, add salt and pepper to the food.

8. Make your Caprese salad into a lunchtime meal by adding grilled chicken to it.

Curry with eggplant and chickpeas

Ingredients
1 sliced tiny eggplant
1 can (15 ounces) washed and drained chickpeas
1 cup chopped tomatoes, salt-free from a can;
a quarter cup of light coconut milk;
low-sodium curry powder or paste, if available;

cooking with olive oil;
Salt and pepper to taste;

Instructions

1. In a pan over medium heat, warm the olive oil.

2. When the chopped eggplant begins to soften, add it and continue to sauté.

3. Add the chickpeas, chopped tomatoes, light coconut milk, and curry paste or powder while adjusting the heat to your preference.

4. Simmer the eggplant for 10 to 15 minutes, or until it is soft.

5. To taste, add salt and pepper to the food.

6. For a tasty and filling meal, serve your cooked brown rice or quinoa with your eggplant and chickpea curry.

Quinoa Salad Inspired by Greece

Ingredients
1 serving of cooked quinoa;
1/2 cup diced cucumbers;
1/2 cup diced red bell peppers
1/4 cup chopped red onion
pitted and sliced Kalamata olives; and
crumbled low-fat feta cheese, if desired.
- Greek dressing (preferably low-sodium)
- To taste, salt and pepper

Instructions
1. Cucumber, red bell pepper, and red onion dices, cooked quinoa, and mix in a bowl.

2. For more taste, use crumbled feta cheese and Kalamata olives.

3. Pour on some Greek dressing to give it a genuine flavor.

4. To taste, add salt and pepper to the food.

5. Serve your Greek-inspired quinoa salad as a light and filling lunch by tossing everything together.

Quinoa bowl with turkey and cranberries

Ingredients
1 serving of cooked quinoa;
4 slices of low-sodium roasted turkey breast;
one-fourth cup of unsweetened cranberry sauce;
optional 1/4 cup of chopped pecans;
salt and pepper to taste

Instructions
1. Slices of roasted turkey, cooked quinoa, and cranberry sauce should all be combined in a dish.

2. If preferred, add chopped pecans for a delicious crunch.

3. To taste, add salt and pepper to the food.

4. As a festive and healthy meal, serve your quinoa dish with turkey and cranberries.

White bean and spinach soup

Ingredients
1 can (15 ounces) of washed and drained white beans (cannellini or navy beans)
4 cups of vegetable broth low in salt
Two cups of new spinach leaves
1/2 cup chopped carrots
1/2 cup diced celery
One-half teaspoon dried basil
To taste; salt and pepper

Instructions
1. White beans, low-sodium vegetable broth, fresh spinach leaves, chopped carrots, diced celery, dried basil, salt, and pepper should all be combined in a big saucepan.

2. The mixture should be brought to a boil before being simmered for 20 to 25 minutes,

depending on how tender you want your veggies to be.

3. Serve your spinach and white bean soup as a filling and cozy meal after adjusting the flavor as necessary.

Tuna salad from the Mediterranean

Ingredients
1 can (5 ounces) of drained water-packed tuna;
1/2 cup diced cucumbers;
1/2 cup diced tomatoes;
1/4 cup chopped red onion;
pitted and sliced Kalamata olives;
garnishing with fresh parsley;
low-sodium lemon juice and olive oil for the dressing;
salt and pepper to taste

Instructions
1. The tuna, chopped cucumber, diced tomatoes, and diced red onion should all be combined in a bowl.

2. For more taste, include Kalamata olives.

3. For dressing, drizzle with a concoction of olive oil and lemon juice.

4. To taste, add salt and pepper to the food.

5. Add fresh parsley as a garnish.

6. Serve your Mediterranean tuna salad as a light and protein-packed lunch by tossing everything together.

Chicken Breast Stuffed with Mushrooms and Spinach

Ingredients
a single skinless, boneless chicken breast;
one cup of new spinach leaves;
a serving of sliced mushrooms;
one-fourth cup diced onion;
cooking with olive oil;
salt and pepper to taste;

Instructions

1. Set your oven's temperature to 375°F (190°C).

2. A little bit of olive oil in a pan on medium heat

3. Sauté the mushrooms until tender after adding the chopped onion.

4. Create a pocket by laying the chicken breast flat and cutting a horizontal split through it.

5. Sprinkle a little salt and pepper in the pocket.

6. Place the sautéed mushroom and onion mixture in the pocket, along with some fresh spinach leaves.

7. If necessary, use toothpicks to close the pocket.

8. An oven-safe pan with a little additional olive oil was heated over medium-high heat.

9. The packed chicken breast should be gently browned after being seared for 2 to 3 minutes on each side.

10. When the chicken is fully done, place the pan in the preheated oven and bake for 15-20 minutes.

11. As a tasty and healthy meal, serve chicken breast packed with mushrooms and spinach.

Black bean and quinoa salad

Ingredients
1 serving of cooked quinoa;
1 can (15 ounces) rinsed and drained black beans;
1 cup fresh or frozen corn kernels;
1/4 cup red bell peppers, diced; garnishment of fresh cilantro;
low-sodium olive oil and
lime juice for the dressing
salt and pepper to taste

Instructions

1. The cooked quinoa, black beans, corn, and red bell pepper cubes should all be combined in a dish.

2. For dressing, drizzle with a concoction of lime juice and olive oil.

3. To taste, add salt and pepper to the food.

4. Add fresh cilantro as a garnish.

5. Serve your quinoa and black bean salad as a filling and savory lunch by tossing everything together.

Salmon with spinach salad

Ingredients
1 salmon filet, grilled or baked
Two cups of new spinach leaves;
a serving of sliced strawberries; an optional
1/4 cup of chopped pecans;

balsamic vinaigrette dressing (low-sodium, if desired);
salt and pepper to taste

Instructions

1. Place the fresh spinach leaves in a large salad bowl.

2. Top with the grilled or baked salmon filet.

3. Add sliced strawberries and chopped pecans (if preferred).

4. For taste, drizzle with balsamic vinaigrette dressing.

5. To taste, add salt and pepper to the food.

6. Serve your spinach and salmon salad as a healthy and antioxidant-rich meal.

Curry with sweet potatoes and lentils

Ingredients

cooked green or brown lentils,
1 cup or 2 cups of sweet potatoes, diced;
one (15-ounce) can of diced tomatoes without salt;
a quarter cup of light coconut milk;
low-sodium curry powder or paste, if available;
cooking with olive oil; and
salt and pepper.

Instructions

1. In a big saucepan, warm up the olive oil over medium heat.

2. Sweet potatoes that have been diced should be added and sautéed until they soften.

3. Add the cooked lentils, light coconut milk, chopped tomatoes, and curry powder or paste after adjusting the spice level to your preference.

4. Sweet potatoes should be soft after 15 to 20 minutes of simmering.

5. To taste, add salt and pepper to the food.

6. Serve your curry made with sweet potatoes and lentils as a savory and filling meal.

Fajita bowl with chicken and vegetables

Ingredients
a single skinless, boneless chicken breast;
1 cup of mixed veggies for fajitas, such as bell peppers and onions;
one cup of cooked brown rice;
cooking with olive oil;
a low-sodium fajita spice blend, if you'd like
To taste, salt and pepper

Instructions
1. Salt, pepper, and fajita spice mix are used to season the chicken breast.

2. In a pan, heat the olive oil over medium-high heat.

3. The chicken breast should be cooked for 4-5 minutes on each side, or until done.

4. In a separate skillet, sauté the mixed fajita veggies until they are soft while the chicken cooks.

5. Cut the chicken breast into slices.

6. Cooked brown rice and sautéed faj in a bowl as well as sliced chicken and veggies.

7. Serve your fajita bowl of chicken and vegetables as a wonderful and filling meal.

Mediterranean Quinoa Bowl

Ingredients
1/2 cup sliced cucumber,
1/2 cup diced tomatoes, and
1 cup cooked quinoa;
one-fourth cup of sliced black olives
- A quarter cup of crumbled low-fat feta cheese;
- Fresh basil leaves for garnish;
- Extra-virgin olive oil and low-sodium balsamic vinegar for dressing;

- To taste, salt and pepper

Instructions

1. Place the cooked quinoa, chopped cucumber, diced tomatoes, black olive slices, and feta cheese in a bowl.

2. Dress with a drizzle of a dressing made of olive oil and balsamic vinegar.

3. To taste, add salt and pepper to the dish.

4. Add fresh basil leaves as a garnish.

5. Combine all of the ingredients, then serve your Mediterranean quinoa bowl as a light and protein-packed lunch.

Broccoli and White Bean Soup

Ingredients

2 cups broccoli florets;
1 can (15 ounces) of washed and drained white beans (cannellini or navy beans);

1/2 cup chopped onion;

4 cups low-sodium vegetable broth;

1/2 teaspoon dried thyme; and,

To taste, salt and pepper.

Instructions

1. Combine the white beans, low-sodium vegetable broth, chopped onion, dried thyme, salt, and pepper in a big saucepan with the broccoli florets.

2. After the mixture comes to a boil, turn the heat down to low and let the stew simmer for 20 to 25 minutes, or until the broccoli is soft.

3. Puree the soup using an immersion blender until it is smooth. Alternately, gently add the soup in stages to a blender and process until smooth.

4. Serve your broccoli and white bean soup as a hearty and nourishing meal after adjusting the flavor as necessary.

Tofu with avocado salad

Ingredients

A diced 1/2 brick of firm tofu;
a sliced, half-ripe avocado
2 cups of mixed greens, such as arugula and baby spinach.
Halved cherry tomatoes
Olive oil for dressing (optional), with
a drizzle of lemon juice
To taste, salt and pepper

Instructions

1. Place the cubed tofu, avocado slices, mixed greens, and cherry tomatoes in a bowl.

2. To add flavor, drizzle with lemon juice and olive oil (if preferred).

3. To taste, add salt and pepper to the dish.

4. Combine all of the ingredients, then serve your tofu and avocado salad as a healthy and revitalizing lunch.

Curry made with cauliflower and chickpeas

Ingredients
2 cups of cauliflower
1 can (15 ounces) of washed and drained chickpeas
1 cup chopped tomatoes, salt-free from a can;
a quarter cup of light coconut milk
low-sodium curry powder or paste, if available;
cooking with olive oil
To taste, salt and pepper

Instructions
1. In a pan over medium heat, warm the olive oil.

2. Include the cauliflower florets and cook them in the pan until they begin to soften.

3. Add the curry powder or paste, chickpeas, chopped tomatoes, light coconut milk, and curry paste (tune the amount of heat to your liking).

4. Simmer the cauliflower for 10 to 15 minutes, or until it is soft.

5. To taste, add salt and pepper to the food.

6. For a tasty and filling meal, serve your cooked brown rice or quinoa with your cauliflower and chickpea curry.

Turkey and Cranberry Salad

Ingredients
1 cup low-sodium cooked and diced turkey breast
1/2 cup dried cranberries (optionally without sugar)
- Optional 1/4 cup of chopped pecans mixed greens, such as arugula and baby spinach.
low-sodium balsamic vinaigrette dressing, if desired;
To taste, salt and pepper

Instructions

1. Place cooked, diced turkey breast, dried cranberries, and optional chopped pecans in a bowl.

2. Combine the ingredients with mixed greens.

3. To add flavor, drizzle with balsamic vinaigrette dressing.

4. To taste, add salt and pepper to the dish.

5. Make a spectacular meal out of your turkey and cranberry salad.

Lentil and Veggie Stir-Fry

Ingredients
2 cups combined, stirred with
1 cup of cooked green or brown lentils
low-sodium stir-fry sauce;
fried veggies (such as bell peppers, snap peas, and carrots);
1 cup cooked quinoa or brown rice
Cooking with olive oil

To taste, salt and pepper

Instructions

1. In a large skillet or wok, heat the olive oil over medium-high heat.

2. Include the mixed stir-fry veggies and continue to stir-fry until the vegetables begin to soften.

3. Add the stir-fry sauce and cooked lentils.

4. Continue to cook for an additional 1-2 minutes to fully reheat.

5. Spoon the cooked brown rice or quinoa over the lentil and vegetable stir-fry.

6. To taste, add salt and pepper.

7. Indulge in a short and tasty meal.

Tomato Basil Quinoa Salad

Ingredients
1 cup quinoa that has been cooked;
1 cup chopped tomatoes
Tear some fresh basil leaves.
- Low-sodium balsamic vinaigrette dressing, if desired;
- Optional drizzle of olive oil;
- To taste, salt and pepper

Instructions
1. Combine the cooked quinoa, chopped tomatoes, and freshly torn basil leaves in a dish.

2. For taste, drizzle with balsamic vinaigrette dressing.

3. If preferred, add a drizzle of olive oil.

4. To taste, add salt and pepper to the dish.

5. Combine all of the ingredients, then serve your tomato basil quinoa salad as a healthy and revitalizing meal.

Spinach and Chickpea Wrap

Ingredients
One whole-wheat tortilla and one cup of new spinach leaves
1/2 cup mashed chickpeas
1/4 cup cucumbers, diced
Hummus for dipping
- To taste, salt and pepper

Instructions
1. The whole-grain tortilla should be laid out flat on a tidy surface.

2. Cover the tortilla with a uniform coating of hummus.

3. Scatter some new spinach leaves over the hummus.

4. Cover the spinach with mashed chickpeas.

5. Include cucumber dice.

6. To taste, add salt and pepper.

7. After securely rolling the wrap, cut it in half.

8. Offer your chickpea and spinach wrap as a quick and wholesome lunch.

Quinoa and Grilled Veggie Bowl

Ingredients
Assorted grilled veggies, such as zucchini, bell peppers, and eggplant
1 cup cooked quinoa;
olive oil for drizzling (optional)
- Fresh lemon juice for dripping
- To taste, salt and pepper

Instructions
1. Grill the veggies of your choosing until they are soft and just beginning to brown.

2. Place the cooked quinoa and grilled veggies in a dish.

3. For taste, drizzle with extra virgin olive oil and fresh lemon juice.

4. To taste, add salt and pepper to the dish.

5. Combine everything and serve your quinoa and grilled vegetable bowl as a savory and filling meal.

Foil packets with salmon and asparagus

Ingredients
lemon slices,
asparagus stalks, and
one salmon filet
Dill for taste, fresh
A drizzle of olive oil
Salt and pepper to taste

Instructions
1. Set the oven's temperature to 375°F (190°C).

2. Lay the salmon filet out on a sheet of foil.

3. Place lemon slices and asparagus spears around the fish.

4. Add some freshly chopped dill and some olive oil.

5. To taste, add salt and pepper to the food.

6. Seal the foil's edges as you fold it into a bundle.

7. Bake the salmon in the preheated oven for 15-20 minutes, or until it is well done.

8. Offer the foil package of salmon and asparagus as a tasty and light lunch.

Quinoa and Veggie Stir-Fry

Ingredients
2 cups of mixed stir-fry veggies, such as broccoli, bell peppers, and snap peas
1 cup of cooked quinoa
low-sodium sauce for stir-fries

Cooking with olive oil
To taste, salt and pepper

Instructions

1. In a large skillet or wok, heat the olive oil over medium-high heat.

2. Include the mixed stir-fry veggies and continue to stir-fry until the vegetables begin to soften.

3. Combine the stir-fry sauce and cooked quinoa.

4. Continue to cook for an additional 1-2 minutes to fully reheat.

5. Offer the stir-fried quinoa and vegetables as a fast and filling meal.

6. To taste, add salt and pepper.

Caprese quinoa salad

Ingredients

1 cup of cooked quinoa

Halved cherry tomatoes

Balls of fresh mozzarella cheese

Tear some fresh basil leaves

low-sodium balsamic vinaigrette dressing, if desired

Optional drizzle of olive oil

To taste, salt and pepper

Instructions

1. Place the prepared quinoa, cherry tomatoes, fresh mozzarella cheese balls, and freshly torn basil leaves in a bowl.

2. For taste, drizzle with balsamic vinaigrette dressing.

3. If preferred, add a drizzle of olive oil.

4. To taste, add salt and pepper to the dish.

5. Combine all of the ingredients, then serve your Caprese quinoa salad as a filling lunch.

These lunch recipes offer a range of tastes and options to broaden your selection of gastritis-friendly foods. While taking good care of your tummy, enjoy your meals!

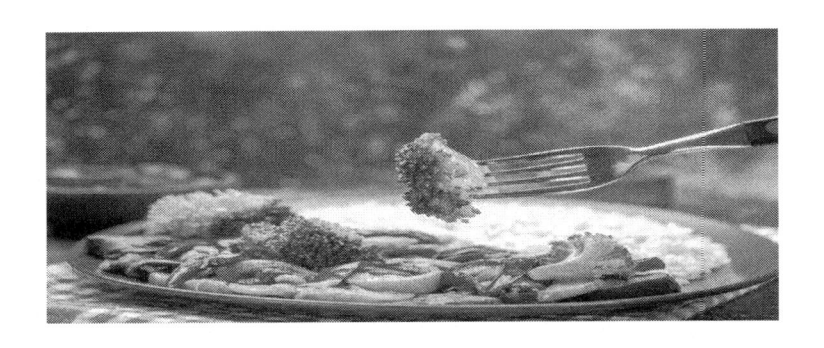

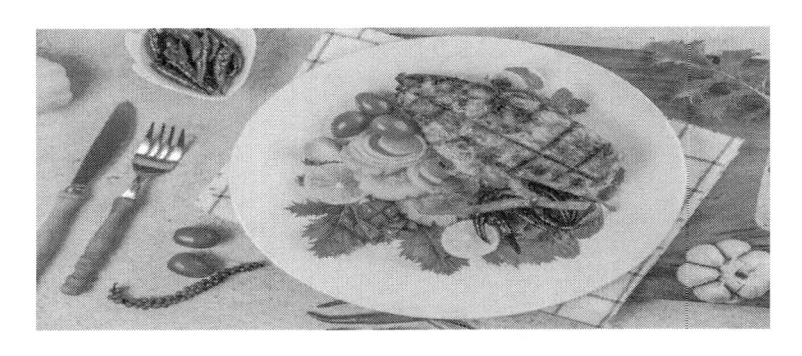

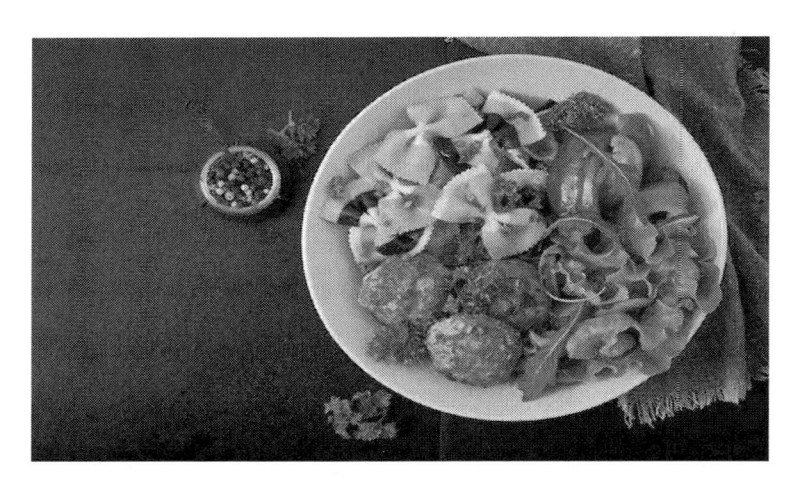

CHAPTER SIX

Recipes for a Gastritis-Friendly Dinner

Salmon Baked with Lemon and Herbs

Ingredients
Fresh dill or parsley;
2 salmon filets
1 lemon, thinly sliced
To taste, salt and pepper.

Instructions
1. Set the oven's temperature to 375°F (190°C).

2. Arrange the salmon filets on a parchment-lined baking pan.

3. Add some olive oil and salt and pepper to the fish.

4. Top each filet with lemon slices and fresh dill or parsley.

5. Bake the salmon for 15 to 20 minutes, or until it flakes easily.

6. Include a side of sautéed green beans or asparagus along with the steaming white rice.

Stir-fry with quinoa and vegetables

Ingredients
2 cups of water
1 cup of blanched and drained broccoli florets;
1 cup sliced red, yellow, or green bell peppers
1 cup thinly sliced carrots;
1 cup thinly sliced zucchini;
2 cloves of minced garlic
low-sodium tamari or soy sauce
Sesame seed oil,
To taste, salt, and pepper

Instructions
1. Bring water to a boil in a medium saucepan, then stir in the quinoa. Once quinoa is frothy,

reduce heat, cover, and cook for 15 to 20 minutes.

2. Heat a small quantity of sesame oil over medium-high heat in a big pan or wok.

3. Stir-fry the minced garlic for around 30 seconds.

4. Add the veggies, slice them, and stir-fry for 5 to 7 minutes, or until they are crisp-tender.

5. Add the cooked quinoa to the pan and combine with the low-sodium soy sauce.

6. To taste, add salt and pepper.

7. Serve immediately as a filling stir-fry.

Chicken Soup with Ginger and Turmeric

Ingredients
2 skinless, boneless breasts of chicken;
1 chopped onion;

2 minced garlic cloves;

1 inch of grated fresh ginger;

1 teaspoon of crushed turmeric

6 cups of low-sodium chicken broth,

1 cup of chopped carrots,

1 cup of chopped celery,

salt to taste, and

optionally, fresh cilantro

Instructions

1. Heat a little olive oil in a big saucepan over medium heat. Add grated ginger, minced garlic, and onion. Sauté until aromatic for a few minutes.

2. Stir for another minute after adding the ground turmeric.

3. Fill the saucepan with chicken breasts, chicken stock, carrots, and celery. Heat till boiling, then lower to a simmer and cover.

4. Cook the chicken for 20 to 25 minutes, or until it is fully done.

5. Take the chicken out of the saucepan, shred it with a fork, and put it back in.

6. Add salt and pepper to taste and season the soup.

7. If preferred, sprinkle with fresh cilantro and serve hot.

Baked Chicken and Veggie Casserole

Ingredients
2 skinless, boneless breasts of chicken;
two cups of sliced zucchini;
two cups of sliced red, yellow, or green bell peppers
One cup of sliced tomatoes and
2 minced garlic cloves
1 teaspoon each of dried basil and oregano
Oil of olives:
To taste, salt, and pepper

Instructions

1. Set the oven's temperature to 375°F (190°C).

2. Arrange the cut veggies around the chicken breasts in a baking dish.

3. Olive oil should be drizzled over everything before minced garlic, dried basil, and dried oregano are added.

4. To taste, add salt and pepper to the dish.

5. Bake the dish for 25 to 30 minutes with the foil covering. Once the chicken is cooked through and the veggies are soft, remove the lid and continue baking for an additional 10–15 minutes.

6. Present hot.

Vegetable and Lentil Soup

Ingredients
1 cup washed and drained dry green or brown lentils;

6 cups low-sodium vegetable broth;
1 chopped onion;
2 chopped carrots;
2 chopped celery stalks
2 minced garlic cloves;
1 bay leaf;
1 teaspoon dry thyme; and olive oil;
to taste; salt and pepper.

Instructions

1. Heat a little olive oil in a big saucepan over medium heat. Add the chopped celery, carrots, onion, and garlic. Several minutes of sautéing will soften.

2. Fill the saucepan with the lentils, vegetable broth, dried thyme, and bay leaf. Heat till boiling, then lower to a simmer and cover.

3. Cook the lentils for 25 to 30 minutes, or until they are soft.

4. Take out the bay leaf and add salt and pepper to taste to the soup.

5. Serve hot as a hearty vegetable and lentil soup.

Grilled turkey or chicken skewers

Ingredients
2 chicken or turkey breasts, cut into cubes, that are boneless and skinless
Plum tomatoes and red onion pieces
pieces of bell pepper
Lemon juice with olive oil
dried thyme,
to taste, salt, and pepper

Instructions
1. To create a marinade, combine olive oil, lemon juice, dried rosemary, salt, and pepper in a basin.

2. Alternate cherry tomatoes, bell peppers, and red onion pieces with the cubes of chicken or turkey as you thread them onto skewers.

3. Apply the marinade to the skewers.

4. Preheat a grill or grill pan to medium-high heat. Cook the kebabs, rotating them every few minutes, for approximately 10 to 15 minutes, or until the meat is well cooked.

5. Serve with brown rice or quinoa that has been steam-cooked.

Vegetable and Tofu Stir-Fry

Ingredients
1 block of diced firm tofu
2 cups of broccoli florets;
1 cup sliced red, yellow, or green bell peppers; and
1 serving of sliced mushrooms
2 minced garlic cloves
low-sodium tamari or soy sauce
Sesame seed oil,
To taste, salt, and pepper

Instructions

1. After pressing the tofu to get rid of extra moisture, chop it into cubes.

2. Heat a small quantity of sesame oil over medium-high heat in a big pan or wok.

3. Stir-fry the minced garlic for around 30 seconds.

4. Include the tofu cubes and stir-fry them until just starting to brown.

5. Add the mushrooms, broccoli, and bell peppers to the pan and stir-fry for 5 to 7 minutes, or until the veggies are crisp-tender.

6. Pour tamari or low-sodium soy sauce over the stir-fry and combine everything.

7. To taste, add salt and pepper to the dish.

8. Spoon warm brown rice on top.

Roasted Vegetable Medley

Ingredients
- Olive oil;
- Fresh thyme leaves;
- A variety of veggies (such as carrots, zucchini, bell peppers, and cherry tomatoes)
Balsamic vinaigrette,
to taste, salt and pepper

Instructions
1. Set the oven's temperature to 400°F (200°C).

2. Chop up the veggies, then spread them out on a baking sheet.

3. Drizzle balsamic vinegar and olive oil over the veggies. Sprinkle salt, pepper, and new thyme leaves.

4. Stir the veggies to ensure that the spice is distributed evenly.

5. Roast the veggies in the oven for 20 to 25 minutes, or until they are soft and have begun to caramelize.

6. Offer it as a tasty and colorful side dish.

Cod Baked in Lemon and Herbs

Ingredients
1 lemon, finely sliced;
2 fish filets; fresh parsley;
olive oil (to taste);
salt and pepper.

Instructions
1. Set the oven's temperature to 375°F (190°C).

2. Arrange the fish filets on a parchment-lined baking sheet.

3. Add some olive oil and salt and pepper to the fish.

4. Top each filet with lemon slices and fresh parsley.

5. Bake the fish for 15 to 20 minutes, or until it flakes easily.

6. Arrange quinoa and cooked asparagus on the side.

Peppers Stuffed with Sweet Potato and Black Beans

Ingredients
1 can black beans, drained and rinsed;
1 cup diced sweet potatoes, roasted;
1 cup diced tomatoes;
1 teaspoon each of powdered cumin and chili powder
4 bell peppers, split and seeds removed;
2 cups cooked quinoa;
Salt and pepper to taste

Instructions
1. Set the oven's temperature to 375°F (190°C).

2. Combine cooked quinoa, black beans, sweet potatoes that have been roasted, chopped tomatoes, cumin, chili powder, salt, and pepper in a big bowl.

3. Stuff the quinoa and bean mixture into each half of a bell pepper.

4. Put the peppers in a baking tray and cover with foil.

5. Bake the peppers for 30-35 minutes, or until they are soft.

6. Toss with a dab of tahini sauce or a dollop of Greek yogurt.

Meatballs made with turkey and vegetables

Ingredients
1/2 cup finely chopped zucchini and carrots, plus 1 pound of ground turkey;
1/4 cups minced spinach;

2 minced garlic cloves
1 tsp. dried oregano
To taste-test salt and pepper
Olive oil for baking

Instructions

1. Set the oven's temperature to 375°F (190°C).

2. Combine the ground turkey with the grated zucchini, carrots, spinach, minced garlic, dried oregano, salt, and pepper in a large bowl.

3. Scoop out meatballs from the mixture and set them on a baking sheet covered with parchment paper.

4. Lightly brush some olive oil on the meatballs.

5. Bake the meatballs for 20 to 25 minutes, or until they are well cooked and browned.

6. Include quinoa and steaming green beans on the side.

Mashable cauliflower with chives and garlic

Ingredients
1 cauliflower head, separated into florets
2 minced garlic cloves;
2 freshly cut chives
Oil of olives:
To taste, salt and pepper

Instructions
1. To make the cauliflower florets soft, steam them.

2. Combine the steamed cauliflower, minced garlic, extra virgin olive oil, salt, and pepper in a food processor and pulse until smooth.

3. Place the mashed cauliflower on a serving platter and top with freshly cut chives.

4. Used as a cozy side dish that is creamy.

Lentil and Veggie Stir-Fry

Ingredients

2 cups of water,

2 cups of mixed veggies (broccoli, bell peppers, carrots),

1 cup of washed and drained green or brown lentils,

2 cloves of minced garlic, and

low-sodium soy sauce or tamari.

Sesame seed oil:

To taste, salt, and pepper

Instructions

1. Bring water to a boil in a medium saucepan, then add lentils. Once lentils are cooked, reduce heat, cover, and simmer for 15 to 20 minutes.

2. Heat a small quantity of sesame oil over medium-high heat in a big pan or wok.

3. Stir-fry the minced garlic for around 30 seconds.

4. Stir-fry the mixed veggies for 5-7 minutes, or until they are tender-crisp.

5. Pour low-sodium soy sauce or tamari over the cooked lentils in the pan and combine everything.

6. To taste, add salt and pepper.

7. Serve hot as a filling stir-fry with lentils and vegetables.

Baked sweet potato fries

Ingredients
2 big, cut-up sweet potatoes
Paprika,
olive oil, and
Ground garlic
To taste, salt and pepper

Instructions
1. Set the oven's temperature to 425°F (220°C).

2. Place sweet potato fries in a big bowl and add olive oil, paprika, garlic powder, salt, and pepper.

3. Arrange the fries on a parchment-lined baking sheet.

4. Bake the fries in the oven for 20 to 25 minutes, rotating them halfway through, or until they are crispy and browned.

5. Used as a tasty and wholesome side dish.

Quinoa with roasted vegetables and herbs

Ingredients
2 cups low-sodium vegetable broth; assorted roasted veggies (such as bell peppers, zucchini, and cherry tomatoes)
1 cup washed and drained quinoa,
fresh parsley, and basil
Oil of olives:
balsamic vinegar
Taste-tested salt and pepper

Instructions

1. Bring the vegetable broth to a boil in a saucepan before adding the quinoa. Once quinoa is frothy, reduce heat, cover, and cook for 15 to 20 minutes.

2. Add a sprinkle of olive oil to your chosen veggies and roast them until they are soft.

3. Mix the quinoa that has been cooked with the roasted veggies.

4. Top the dish with fresh basil and parsley, and drizzle it with olive oil and balsamic vinegar.

5. To taste, add salt and pepper to the food.

6. Offer a tasty and colorful meal.

Ginger and carrot soup

Ingredients
1 onion, diced;

6 big carrots, peeled and chopped;
2 cloves of minced garlic;
a grated 1-inch piece of fresh ginger
Olive oil and
four cups of low-sodium vegetable broth—
coriander seeds
To taste, salt and pepper.

Instructions

1. Heat a little olive oil in a big saucepan over medium heat. Add the minced garlic, grated ginger, and diced onion. Sauté until aromatic for a few minutes.

2. Stir in the chopped carrots for a few more minutes.

3. Add the veggie broth and heat through. Simmer for 20 to 25 minutes, covered, or until the carrots are tender.

4. Puree the soup using an immersion blender until it is smooth. Alternately, add the soup in batches to a blender.

5. Add salt, pepper, and ground coriander to taste.

6. Serve hot as a soothing soup made with ginger and carrots.

Portobello Mushrooms Stuffed with Turkey and Spinach

Ingredients
2 cups chopped fresh spinach;
4 big Portobello mushrooms;
1 pound mince turkey; and
1/2 cup diced tomatoes
2 minced garlic cloves
Italian spices
Oil of olives:
To taste, salt and pepper

Instructions
1. Set the oven's temperature to 375°F (190°C).

2. Sprinkle salt and pepper over the Portobello mushrooms after brushing them with olive oil. On a baking sheet, put them.

3. Brown the ground turkey in a pan over medium heat. Remove any extra fat.

4. Fill the pan with diced tomatoes, chopped spinach, minced garlic, and Italian spice. Sauté for a few minutes, stirring often, just until the spinach wilts.

5. Place a portion of the turkey and spinach mixture into each Portobello mushroom cap.

6. Bake the mushrooms for 20 to 25 minutes, or until they are soft.

7. Serve warm for a flavorful and filling supper.

Grilled Shrimp Skewers with Lemon and Herbs

Ingredients

1 pound of big shrimp that have been peeled and deveined.
Fresh rosemary or thyme
Salt and pepper to taste;
olive oil

Instructions

1. Set the grill to a medium-high temperature.

2. Combine fresh lemon juice, fresh thyme or rosemary, olive oil, salt, and pepper in a dish and use to marinade the shrimp.

3. Skewer the shrimp that have been marinated.

4. Grill the shrimp skewers for a total of 2 to 3 minutes on each side, or until they are opaque and pink.

5. Provide quinoa or a green salad as a side dish.

Roasted butternut squash soup

Ingredients

1 cubed butternut squash, peeled, seeded, and diced;
1 chopped onion
2 minced garlic cloves
Olive oil,
fresh sage leaves, and
Low-sodium vegetable broth;
Taste-tested salt and pepper

Instructions

1. Set the oven's temperature to 375°F (190°C).

2. Combine diced butternut squash with sage leaves and olive oil. Roast in the oven until cooked through and browned.

3. Saute chopped onion and minced garlic in olive oil in a big saucepan till tender.

4. Include the roasted butternut squash in the saucepan and cover it with vegetable broth.

5. Allow to simmer for 15 to 20 minutes.

6. Puree the soup using an immersion blender until it is smooth. To taste, add salt and pepper to the food.

7. Serve hot as a hearty soup made from roasted butternut squash.

Chicken Breast Stuffed with Spinach and Feta

Ingredients
2 skinless, boneless chicken breasts,
fresh spinach, and
crumbled feta cheese
Lemon zest,
olive oil, and
salt and pepper to taste.

Instructions
1. Set the oven's temperature to 375°F (190°C).

2. Create a pocket in the chicken breasts by making a horizontal incision in them.

3. Add feta cheese crumbles and fresh spinach leaves to each chicken breast.

4. Add a drizzle of olive oil and season with salt and pepper.

5. Bake the chicken for 25 to 30 minutes, or until fully done.

6. Provide quinoa or broccoli as a side dish.

Baked turkey and vegetable casserole

Ingredients
2 cups of chopped mixed veggies, such as carrots, bell peppers, and zucchini;
1 pound of ground turkey;
1 chopped onion;
2 minced garlic cloves
Oil of olives:
paprika
To taste, salt and pepper.

Instructions

1. Set the oven's temperature to 375°F (190°C).

2. Heat a little olive oil in a pan over medium-high heat. Add minced garlic and onion, chopped. until softened, sauté.

3. Add the turkey ground and heat it until it is browned. Remove any extra fat.

4. Arrange the cooked turkey, mixed veggies, paprika, salt, and pepper in a baking dish.

5. Bake the veggies for 25 to 30 minutes, or until they are soft.

6. Serve the dish hot to provide comfort.

Bell Peppers Stuffed with Quinoa

Ingredients
1 cup cooked quinoa,
1 cup diced tomatoes,
1 cup cooked black beans, and
4 bell peppers with the tops and seeds removed.

- Olive oil
- 1 teaspoon ground cumin
- To taste, salt and pepper

Instructions

1. Set the oven's temperature to 375°F (190°C).

2. Combine cooked quinoa, diced tomatoes, black beans, corn, cumin powder, a drizzle of olive oil, salt, and pepper in a big bowl.

3. Fill the quinoa mixture into each bell pepper.

4. Bake the filled peppers for 30-35 minutes, or until they are soft. Place them in a baking dish, cover with foil, and bake.

5. Top heated dishes with fresh cilantro or a dollop of Greek yogurt.

Lemon Herb Grilled Chicken

Ingredients
2 skinless, boneless breasts of chicken;

Lemonade just squeezed;
fresh herbs (such as thyme and rosemary)
Oil of olives;
ground garlic;
to taste; salt and pepper;

Instructions

1. In a bowl, combine the fresh lemon juice, fresh herbs, olive oil, garlic powder, salt, and pepper with the chicken breasts to form a marinade.

2. Set the temperature of your grill to medium-high.

3. Grill the chicken breasts for 6 to 7 minutes on each side, or until done.

4. Arrange roasted sweet potatoes or steamed asparagus on the side.

Vegetable and Brown Rice Stir-Fry

Ingredients

2 cups of mixed veggies, such as broccoli, snap peas, and carrots
1 cup of cooked brown rice;
2 minced garlic cloves
low-sodium tamari or soy sauce
Sesame seed oil:
to taste, salt, and pepper

Instructions

1. Heat a small quantity of sesame oil to medium-high heat in a big skillet or wok.

2. Stir-fry the minced garlic for around 30 seconds.

3. Stir-fry the mixed veggies for 5-7 minutes, or until they are tender-crisp.

4. Pour low-sodium soy sauce or tamari over the cooked brown rice in the pan and combine everything.

5. To taste, add salt and pepper to the food.

6. Serve hot as a filling stir-fry of vegetables and brown rice.

Sweet potatoes baked in the oven with a chickpea and avocado topping

Ingredients
1 can of rinsed and drained chickpeas
1 ripe avocado
2 medium sweet potatoes,
olive oil
Citrus juice
Smoldering paprika
To taste, salt and pepper

Instructions
1. Set the oven's temperature to 400°F (200°C).

2. To make the sweet potatoes soft, prick them with a fork and bake them for 40 to 45 minutes.

3. Combine chickpeas, chopped avocado, lime juice, smoked paprika, salt, and pepper in a bowl, along with a splash of olive oil.

4. When the sweet potatoes have finished cooking, cut them in half and spread the chickpea and avocado mixture on top.

5. Serve hot as a satisfying and nourishing supper.

Tomato and Basil Grilled Cheese Sandwich

Ingredients
slices of low-fat mozzarella cheese,
sliced tomatoes, fresh basil, and
whole-grain bread.
Olive oil (used for grilling).

Instructions
1. Build your sandwich with pieces of low-fat mozzarella cheese, whole-grain bread, tomatoes, and fresh basil.

2. Apply a thin layer of olive oil to the sandwich's outside.

3. In a panini press or on a skillet, grill the sandwich until the cheese is melted and the bread is crisp.

4. Provide a side salad and serve hot.

Lemon-garlic Shrimp Pasta

Ingredients
8 ounces of whole-grain pasta,
1 pound of peeled and deveined shrimp,
2 cloves of chopped garlic, and
fresh lemon juice
Olive oil, fresh parsley, and
To taste, salt and pepper.

Instructions
1. Prepare the whole-grain pasta per the directions on the box, then drain.

2. Warm up the olive oil in a pan over medium heat. Add the minced garlic and cook for 30 seconds or so.

3. Include the shrimp and sauté them in the pan until they are opaque and pink.

4. Toss the cooked pasta and shrimp with some freshly squeezed lemon juice and fresh parsley for decoration.

5. To taste, add salt and pepper to the food. As a tasty shrimp pasta meal, serve hot.

A quinoa bowl with roasted Brussels sprouts

Ingredients
two cups of cooked quinoa,
two cups of roasted
Brussels sprouts, and
one-quarter cup of almonds.
Salt and pepper to taste,
balsamic vinegar, and
olive oil

Instructions
1. Combine cooked quinoa with roasted Brussels sprouts and almonds.

2. Drizzle with balsamic vinegar and olive oil.

3. To taste, add salt and pepper to the dish.

4. Use as a filling and healthy quinoa dish.

Stir-fry with turkey and vegetables

Ingredients
2 cups of mixed veggies, such as broccoli, bell peppers, and snap peas;
1 pound of ground turkey;
2 minced garlic cloves
low-sodium tamari or soy sauce
Sesame seed oil
To taste, salt and pepper.

Instructions
1. Brown the ground turkey in a pan over medium-high heat. Remove any extra fat.

2. Include mixed veggies and minced garlic in the skillet. Vegetables should be stir-fried for 5-7 minutes, or until they are crisp-tender.

3. Add a dab of sesame oil and low-sodium soy sauce or tamari.

4. To taste, add salt and pepper to the dish.

5. Serve hot as a delectable stir-fry with vegetables and turkey.

Sweet potatoes mashed with cinnamon

Ingredients
- 2 huge sweet potatoes, chopped and peeled;
- cinnamon-ground oil of olives;
- salt and pepper to taste;

Instructions
1. Soften the sliced sweet potatoes by boiling or steaming them.

2. Add a dash of olive oil, some ground cinnamon, salt, and pepper to taste, and mash the sweet potatoes.

3. Make it into a hearty side dish.

Grilled Salmon with Lemon and Herbs

Ingredients
Fresh lemon juice;
2 salmon filets
Olive oil,
fresh herbs (such as dill and thyme), and
garlic powder
To taste, salt and pepper

Instructions
1. Set the grill to a medium-high temperature.

2. Season the salmon filets with salt, pepper, fresh lemon juice, fresh herbs, olive oil, and garlic powder.

3. Grill the salmon for four to five minutes on each side, or until it flakes easily.

4. Provide quinoa or green beans as a side dish.

Mediterranean Chickpea Salad

Ingredients
1 can of rinsed and drained chickpeas
Diced cucumber; finely chopped
red onion; pitted and sliced
Kalamata olives;
crumbled feta cheese
Olive oil, fresh parsley,
balsamic vinegar,
taste-tested salt, and pepper

Instructions
1. Combine the chickpeas, feta cheese crumbles, Kalamata olives, cucumber, red onion, cherry tomatoes, and fresh parsley in a big bowl.

2. Drizzle with balsamic vinegar and olive oil.

3. To taste, add salt and pepper to the dish.

4. Combine all of the ingredients.

5. Serve as a light chickpea salad from the Mediterranean.

Salmon baked with dill and lemon

Ingredients
Fresh dill and lemon slices
2 salmon filets
Oil of olives:
To taste, salt and pepper

Instructions
1. Set the oven's temperature to 375°F (190°C).

2. Arrange the salmon filets on a parchment-lined baking pan.

3. Add some olive oil and salt and pepper to the fish.

4. Place thin slices of lemon and fresh dill on top of each filet.

5. Bake the salmon for 15 to 20 minutes, or until it flakes easily.

6. Provide quinoa or broccoli as a side dish.

Zucchini noodles with pesto and cherry tomatoes

Ingredients
Zoodles prepared from zucchini;
halved cherry tomatoes;
homemade or premade pesto sauce
Pine nuts, if desired
Oil of olives:
To taste, salt and pepper

Instructions
1. Slightly warm some olive oil in a pan over medium heat.

2. Include cherry tomatoes and zucchini noodles. Heat through after 2–3 minutes of sautéing.

3. Toss with pine nuts (if using) and pesto sauce.

4. To taste, add salt and pepper to the dish.

5. Used as a tasty and light zucchini noodle meal.

Chicken and rice soup

Ingredients
2 skinless, boneless breasts of chicken
1 cup of cooked brown rice and
a variety of veggies, such as carrots, celery, and peas
Fresh parsley;
low-sodium chicken broth;
to taste; salt and pepper

Instructions

1. Place chicken breasts, mixed veggies, and sufficient low-sodium chicken stock to cover in a big saucepan.

2. Bring to a boil, then lower the heat and simmer the chicken until the desired doneness.

3. Take the chicken out of the saucepan, shred it, and put it back in.

4. Include fresh parsley and cooked brown rice.

5. To taste, add salt and pepper to the food.

6. Make a hearty chicken and rice soup to serve.

Baked Eggplant Parmesan

Ingredients
Cut eggplant;
Marinara sauce without added salt;
Parmesan cheese, grated;
part-skim mozzarella cheese;
dried oregano

Olive oil,

To taste, salt, and pepper

Instructions

1. Set the oven's temperature to 375°F (190°C).

2. Sprinkle salt, pepper, and dried oregano over slices of grilled eggplant before brushing with olive oil.

3. Arrange eggplant pieces, marinara sauce, and mozzarella cheese in layers in a baking dish.

4. Sprinkle grated Parmesan cheese on top.

5. Bake for 30-35 minutes, or until the cheese is bubbling and brown and the eggplant is soft.

6. Put some mixed greens or a green salad on the side.

Stuffed mushrooms with turkey and spinach

Ingredients

Big mushroom caps;
turkey ground up
chopped fresh spinach;
garlic powder
Oil of olives:
to taste, salt, and pepper

Instructions

1. Set the oven's temperature to 375°F (190°C).

2. Cut the mushroom stems off, then arrange the caps on a baking sheet.

3. Brown ground turkey in a skillet with a little olive oil. Remove any extra fat.

4. Add the chopped fresh spinach and season to taste with salt, pepper, and garlic powder.

5. Fill the turkey and spinach mixture into each mushroom cap.

6. Bake the mushrooms for 20 to 25 minutes, or until they are soft.

7. Used as a delicious and filling starter or main dish.

Roasted asparagus and cherry tomato pasta

Ingredients
Trimmed asparagus spears;
whole-grain pasta
Olive oil,
fresh basil leaves,
balsamic vinegar,
salt, and pepper to taste
Halved cherry tomatoes.

Instructions
1. Prepare the whole-grain pasta per the directions on the box, then drain.

2. Roast cherry tomatoes and asparagus spears in olive oil until they are tender.

3. Combine the pasta that has been cooked with the roasted veggies, the basil, and a little balsamic vinegar.

4. To taste, add salt and pepper to the dish.

5. Use as a vibrant and tasty pasta dish.

Bell Peppers Stuffed with Quinoa and Vegetables

Ingredients
1 cup cooked quinoa;
4 bell peppers with the tops and seeds removed;
1 cup of mixed veggies (such as corn, peas, and carrots)
1 can rinsed and drained low-sodium
black beans;
olive oil
Low-sodium
vegetable broth;
To taste; salt and pepper

Instructions

1. Set the oven's temperature to 375°F (190°C).

2. Combine black beans, cooked quinoa, and mixed veggies in a dish.

3. Stuff the quinoa and vegetable mixture into each bell pepper.

4. Put the filled peppers in a baking dish and fill the bottom with some low-sodium vegetable broth.

5. Drizzle with olive oil, and season with salt and pepper.

6. Cover with foil and bake for 30–35 minutes, or until the peppers are cooked.

7. Serve as a healthy and colorful stuffed bell pepper meal.

Lemon Garlic Roasted Chicken Thighs

Ingredients

chicken thighs, bone-in and skinless
Lemonade just squeezed;
fresh rosemary or thyme
Garlic cloves, minced
Oil of olives:
To taste, salt and pepper

Instructions

1. Set the oven's temperature to 375°F (190°C).

2. In a bowl, add fresh lemon juice, minced garlic, olive oil, fresh rosemary or thyme, salt, and pepper.

3. Marinate the chicken thighs in this mixture for around 15-20 minutes.

4. Place the chicken thighs on a baking sheet lined with parchment paper.

5. Roast for 25–30 minutes, or until the chicken is cooked through and golden brown.

6. Provide quinoa or broccoli as a side dish.

Mediterranean Quinoa Salad

Ingredients
2 cups cooked quinoa;
cucumber, diced;
cherry tomatoes, halved;
red onion, finely chopped;
kalamata olives, pitted and sliced;
crumbled feta cheese
Fresh parsley
Olive oil
Red wine
vinegar
Salt and pepper to taste.

Instructions
1. In a large bowl, add cooked quinoa, diced cucumber, split cherry tomatoes, chopped red onion, sliced Kalamata olives, crumbled feta cheese, and fresh parsley.

2. Drizzle with olive oil and red wine vinegar.

3. To taste, add salt and pepper to the dish.

4. Combine all of the ingredients.

5. Present it as a light quinoa salad from the Mediterranean.

Baked chicken and vegetable skewers

Ingredients
Chicken thighs or breast portions;
slices of bell pepper, onion, and zucchini
Paprika, olive oil, and garlic powder
To taste, salt and pepper.

Instructions
1. Set the oven's temperature to 375°F (190°C).

2. Skewers are threaded with bits of chicken and vegetables.

3. Sprinkle salt, pepper, paprika, garlic powder, and olive oil over the skewers.

4. Arrange the skewers on a parchment-lined baking pan.

5. Bake the chicken for 20 to 25 minutes, or until fully done.

6. Present with a fresh salad or a plate of brown rice.

Spaghetti squash with tomato basil sauce

Ingredients
1 spaghetti squash;
homemade or store-bought tomato basil sauce
Fresh basil leaves
Olive oil,
To taste, salt, and pepper

Instructions
1. Set the oven's temperature to 375°F (190°C).

2. Remove the seeds from the spaghetti squash by cutting it in half lengthwise.

3. Arrange the squash halves, cut side up, on a baking sheet.

4. Add salt and pepper, and drizzle with olive oil.

5. Roast the squash for 45 to 50 minutes, or until the threads separate with a fork with ease.

6. Use a fork to scrape the squash strands, then cover with tomato basil sauce and fresh basil.

7. Use as a low-carb substitute for regular spaghetti.

Lettuce wraps with turkey and vegetables

Ingredients
mixed veggies, such as bell peppers, mushrooms, and
water chestnuts
Ground turkey;
low-sodium tamari or soy sauce
- Minced fresh ginger;

- Minced garlic cloves;
- Leaf lettuce, such as iceberg or butter lettuce
Sesame seed oil,
To taste, salt, and pepper

Instructions

1. Brown the ground turkey in a pan over medium heat. Remove any extra fat.

2. Add minced ginger, minced garlic, and mixed veggies to the skillet. Stir-fry the veggies until they are soft.

3. Add a dab of sesame oil and low-sodium soy sauce or tamari.

4. To taste, add salt and pepper to the dish.

5. To make lettuce wraps, spoon the turkey and vegetable mixture into the leaves.

6. Offer a light and healthy lunch.

Lemon Dill Grilled Tilapia

Ingredients
Filets of tilapia with
fresh lemon juice
Olive oil;
fresh dill;
garlic powder
To taste, salt and pepper

Instructions
1. Set the grill to a medium-high temperature.

2. Combine fresh lemon juice, fresh dill, olive oil, garlic powder, salt, and pepper with the tilapia filets to make a marinade.

3. Grill the tilapia for 3 to 4 minutes on each side, or until it flakes with a fork easily.

4. Arrange quinoa or cooked asparagus on the side to serve.

Lentil and Vegetable Soup

Ingredients

1 cup washed and drained dry green or brown lentils;

a variety of veggies, such as carrots, celery, and onions

Fresh thyme or rosemary and low-sodium vegetable broth

Oil of olives:

To taste, salt and pepper

Instructions

1. Heat a little olive oil in a big saucepan over medium heat.

2. Add the mixed veggies and cook until they are tender.

3. Add enough low-sodium vegetable broth to cover the dry lentils, along with fresh thyme or rosemary.

4. Bring to a boil before lowering the heat and simmering the lentils for 25 to 30 minutes, or until they are cooked.

5. To taste, add salt and pepper to the food.

6. Make a wholesome filling with lentil and vegetable soup.

Caprese salad

Ingredients
fresh basil leaves,
fresh tomatoes,
sliced fresh mozzarella cheese,
balsamic vinegar, and
olive oil.
To taste, salt and pepper

Instructions
1. On a platter, alternate tomato and mozzarella slices with fresh basil leaves.

2. Add a drizzle of olive oil and balsamic vinegar.

3. To taste, add salt and pepper to the dish.

4. Use as a tangy and cool Caprese salad.

Stuffed peppers with turkey and quinoa

Ingredients
Ground turkey, with the tops and seeds removed,
bell peppers,
cooked quinoa,
diced tomatoes,
Italian seasoning, and
salt and pepper to taste

Instructions
1. Set the oven's temperature to 375°F (190°C).

2. Brown the ground turkey in a pan over medium-high heat. Remove any extra fat.

3. Fill the pan with the cooked quinoa, diced tomatoes, Italian seasoning, a drop or two of olive oil, salt, and pepper. Stir well to mix.

4. Stuff the turkey and quinoa mixture into each bell pepper.

5. After stuffing the peppers, place them in a baking tray, cover with foil, and bake for 30-35 minutes, or until the peppers are soft.

6. Make a tasty and filling stuffed pepper meal to serve.

Cod Baked with Garlic and Herbs

Ingredients
Cod filets and garlic powder
Fresh herbs (such as thyme and parsley)
Lemon zest,
Olive oil, and
Salt and pepper to taste.

Instructions
1. Set the oven's temperature to 375°F (190°C).

2. Arrange the fish filets on a parchment-lined baking sheet.

3. Combine the fresh herbs, olive oil, lemon zest, salt, and pepper with the minced garlic.

4. Evenly distribute the mixture over the fish filets.

5. Bake the fish for 12 to 15 minutes, or until it flakes easily.

6. Offer quinoa or roasted veggies on the side.

Greek Salad with Grilled Chicken

Ingredients
Grilled breast of chicken
A mixture of greens
- Diced cucumber;
- Halved cherry tomatoes;
- Finely chopped red onion;
- Pitted and sliced Kalamata olives;
- Crumbled feta cheese
Fresh oregano leaves,
red wine vinegar,

olive oil, and salt and pepper to taste.

Instructions

1. Cut the chicken breast into strips after grilling.

2. Combine mixed greens, diced cucumber, cherry tomatoes, red onion, sliced Kalamata olives, and crumbled feta cheese in a big bowl.

3. Add a red wine vinegar and olive oil drizzle.

4. Add salt, pepper, and fresh oregano leaves as desired for seasoning.

5. Mix everything well.

6. Add grilled chicken pieces on top.

7. Use as an enticing and filling Greek salad.

More possibilities for delectable and tummy-friendly dinners are offered by these other gastritis-friendly supper dishes. Enjoy your delicious and relaxing meals!

291

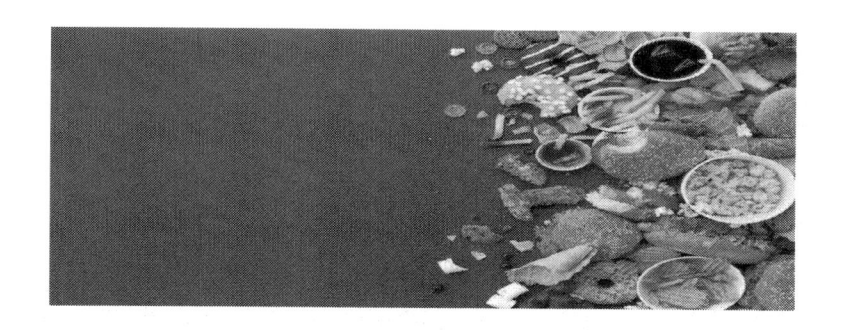

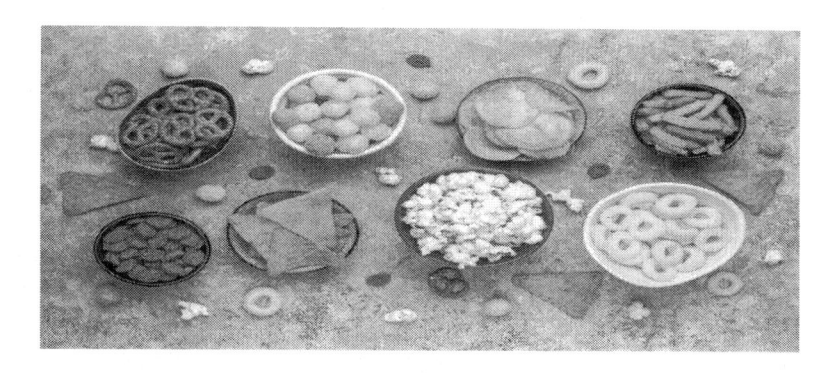

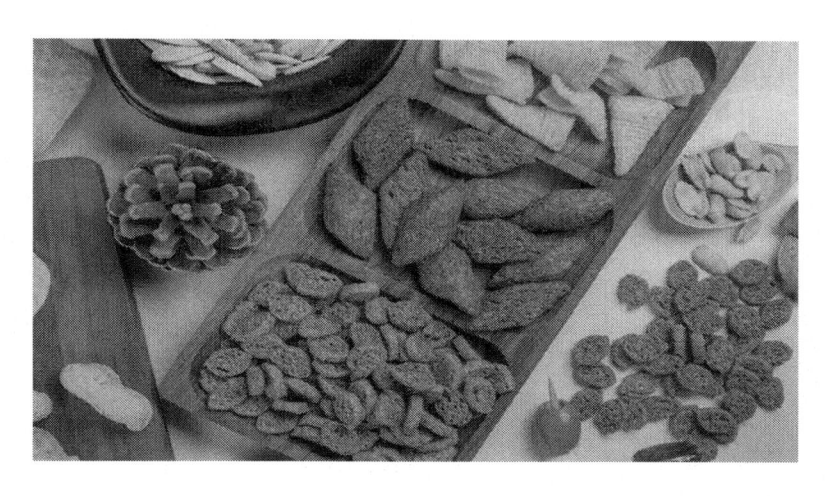

CHAPTER SEVEN

Snack Ideas, Dessert Options and Beverages for Gastritis

Snack Concepts:

Greek yogurt parfait

Ingredient
Unflavored Greek yogurt
Honey Blueberries, strawberries, and other fresh fruit;
Slivered almonds;

Instructions
1. Place Greek yogurt, fresh berries, and a sprinkle of honey in a dish or glass.

2. For more crunch, sprinkle slivered almonds over top.

3. Savor as a rich and filling snack.

Rice Cakes with Avocado

Ingredients
Rice cakes (choose low-sodium varieties).
A mature avocado
Citrus juice,
To taste, salt, and pepper

Instructions
1. Spread rice cakes with mashed avocado.

2. Add salt and pepper, and drizzle with lemon juice.

3. Use as a creamy, crunchy snack.

Almond butter on banana

Ingredients
A ripe banana;
unsweetened almond butter

Instructions

1. Cut up a banana.

2. Spread almond butter on slices of banana.

3. Snack on it for a sweet and nutty treat.

Dessert Selections
Apples Baked with Cinnamon

Ingredients
Sliced apples,
Cinnamon, and (optional) honey

Instructions
1. Set the oven's temperature to 350°F (175°C).

2. Apple slices should be arranged in a baking dish.

3. Add cinnamon and honey (if wanted) as garnishes.

4. Bake the apples for 20 to 25 minutes, or until they are soft.

5. Serve warm as a dessert that is naturally sweet.

Chia Seed Pudding

Ingredients
Chia seeds;
unsweetened almond milk;
delicate berries;
honey, if desired.

1. Combine chia seeds and almond milk in a container or dish using a 1:4 ratio.

2. Stir well and chill for at least several hours or overnight.

3. Add fresh berries and, if preferred, a drizzle of honey on top.

4. Devour as a rich and wholesome dessert.

Freeze-dried banana "ice cream."

Ingredients

Sliced, frozen, ripe bananas;
unsweetened cocoa powder;
vanilla extract, if desired.

Instructions:

1. In a food processor, combine frozen banana slices until creamy.

2. Remix after adding cocoa powder and a little amount of vanilla essence (if desired).

3. To have a firmer texture, freeze for 20 to 30 minutes.

4. Use it to make guilt-free banana "ice cream."

Beverages:
Ginger tea

Ingredients
Sliced fresh ginger root
hot water

honey, if desired

Instructions

1. To make a calming ginger tea, steep fresh ginger slices in hot water.

2. If preferred, add honey for sweetness.

3. Chew gently for better digestion.

Herbal Infusions

Ingredients:
Tea bags with chamomile, peppermint, or fennel;
warm water;

instructions:

1. Prepare herbal tea using tea bags of chamomile, peppermint, or fennel.

2. Permit it to steep for a while.

3. Drink to relax and promote healthy digestion.

Snack Concepts
Sliced Cucumber with Hummus

Ingredients
Thinly sliced cucumbers
Plain, low-fat hummus

Instructions
1. Spread hummus on cucumber slices.

2. Snack on it for a crisp and refreshing treat.

Oatmeal with Banana Slices

(Ingredients)
Plain oatmeal;
sliced ripe banana
Honey (optional) and Cinnamon

Instructions
1. Prepare plain oatmeal according to the directions on the box.

2. Add sliced banana, a dash of cinnamon, and honey (if preferred) to the top.

3. Indulge in a cozy and satiating snack.

Dried Fruits with Mixed Nuts

(Ingredients)
a little amount of mixed nuts, such as almonds and walnuts.
- Dried fruits (such as raisins and apricots).

Instructions:
1. For a balanced snack, combine mixed nuts and dried fruits.

2. Delight in the sweetness and crunchiness of nature.

Dessert Selections
Pears baked with cinnamon and walnuts

Ingredients
ripe pears that have been cored and

half, cinnamon, and chopped walnuts
Honey, if desired.

Instructions

1. Set the oven's temperature to 350°F (175°C).

2. Put a baking dish with pear halves in it.

3. Top with chopped walnuts and cinnamon.

4. If desired, drizzle with honey.

5. Bake the pears for 25 to 30 minutes, or until they are soft.

6. Take pleasure in it as a warm and cozy dessert.

Cool Coconut Rice Pudding

Ingredients
Cooked white rice and coconut milk without added sugar

Maple syrup or agave nectar (optional)
Unsweetened coconut flakes
Kiwi or other fruit slices

Instructions

1. To get the appropriate consistency, combine cooked white rice with unsweetened coconut milk.

2. If desired, add agave nectar or maple syrup to the sweetness.

3. Add sliced kiwis or other fruits and shredded coconut on top.

4. Let cool and consume as a dessert with a tropical flair.

Beverages
Banana and spinach smoothie

Ingredients
a ripe banana.
Fresh spinach leaves;

unsweetened almond milk
Optional ground flaxseed

Instructions
1. Blend almond milk, ripe bananas, and fresh spinach leaves until well combined.

2. If preferred, add ground flaxseed for additional nourishment.

3. Enjoy this calm and nourishing smoothie.

Infusion of peppermint and ginger

Ingredients
A tea bag of peppermint
Slices of fresh ginger;
warm water;

instructions:
1. Brew a peppermint tea bag in hot water with fresh ginger slices.

2. Permit it to steep for a while.

3. Take pleasure in it as a calming and gastrointestinal-friendly beverage.

Snack Concepts:
Cottage cheese and pineapple,

Ingredients
Cottage cheese with less fat;
chunks of fresh pineapple.

Instructions
1. Add some slices of fresh pineapple to a serving of low-fat cottage cheese.

2. Snack on this delicious, creamy treat.

Apple slices with almond butter and cinnamon

Ingredients
Thinly cut apples;
unsweetened almond butter;
ground cinnamon.

Instructions

1. Cover apple slices with almond butter.

2. Add some cinnamon powder on top.

3. Enjoy as a tasty and crispy snack.

Steamed Edamame

Ingredients
Sea salt;
Edamame (young soybeans)

Instructions

1. To make edamame pods delicate, steam them.

2. Add a little amount of sea salt.

3. Enjoy as a filling and high-protein snack.

Dessert Selections
Coconut and berry chia popsicles

Ingredients
Coconut milk without added sugar;
a variety of berries, such as strawberries and blueberries
the chia seed,
honey or agave nectar (optional)

Instructions
1. Combine chia seeds, mixed berries, coconut milk, and sweetener (if preferred) in a blender.

2. Spoon the mixture into popsicle molds and freeze for a firm result.

3. As a cool treat, indulge in these homemade chia popsicles.

Banana and almond ice cream

Ingredients
Sliced, frozen bananas that are ripe
Unsweetened almond butter
Dark chocolate chips (at least 70% cocoa)

Instructions

1. Blend a dollop of almond butter with frozen banana slices until smooth.

2. Add the chocolate chips in the dark.

3. If you'd like a harder texture, freeze.

4. Slurp up like a smooth, somewhat sweet ice cream.

Beverages
Herbal Ginger Lemonade

Ingredients
grated fresh ginger root;
lemon juice
Sparkling water;
honey (optional)

Instructions
1. In a glass, combine freshly grated ginger, lemon juice, and honey (if preferred).

2. Pour sparkling water into the glass.

3. Stir, then sip on the zesty, sparkling beverage.

Iced Mint Tea

Ingredients
ice cubes,
hot water
Fresh mint leaves

Instructions
1. To create mint tea, steep fresh mint leaves in boiling water.

2. Allow it to cool before adding ice.

3. Drink this cooling, calming mint iced tea.

Snack Concepts:
Carrot and hummus dippers

Ingredients
- Baby carrots

- Hummus (choose plain, low-fat variety)

Instructions

1. For a crunchy and creamy snack, dunk baby carrots in hummus.

2. Savor the fusion of tastes and sensations.

Baked sweet potato fries

Ingredients
Fries made with sweet potatoes
Olive oil
- Paprika
- Rosemary, if desired;
- salt and pepper to taste

Instructions
1. Set the oven's temperature to 425°F (220°C).

2. Combine olive oil, paprika, rosemary (if using), salt, and pepper with the sweet potato fries.

3. Bake the fries for 20 to 25 minutes, or until crisp.

4. Enjoy as a wholesome, baked-in snack.

Pumpkin seed-infused trail mix

Ingredients
dried cranberries;
unsweetened coconut flakes
Pumpkin seeds (pepitas) and
chocolate chips, dark (70 percent or more cocoa)

Instructions
1. Combine dark chocolate chips, pumpkin seeds, dried cranberries, and unsweetened coconut flakes.

2. To make a delicious and transportable snack, make your own trail mix.

Dessert Selections
Cinnamon and honey-baked peaches

Ingredients
ripe peaches, pitted and cut in half;
cinnamon;
honey

Instructions
1. Set the oven's temperature to 375°F (190°C).

2. Put the halves of the peaches in a baking dish.

3. Add cinnamon and honey to the surface.

4. Bake the peaches for 20 to 25 minutes, or until they are soft.

5. Devour like a warm dessert that is naturally sweet.

Mango and Banana Smoothie Bowl

Ingredients
Diced ripe mango,
ripe banana, and
unsweetened almond milk

Instructions

1. Blend almond milk, ripe banana, and sliced mango until well combined.

2. Place a bowl with the smoothie inside.

3. Add fresh berries and chia seeds on top.

4. Indulge in a smoothie bowl as a dessert with a tropical theme.

Beverages
Herbal lavender tea

Ingredients

Hot water with dried lavender buds;
lemon wedge, if desired.

Instructions

1. To make a fragrant lavender tea, boil dried lavender buds in hot water.

2. If preferred, add a slice of lemon for added taste.

3. Drink this fragrant beverage to relax.

Watermelon and mint-infused water

Ingredients
Fresh mint leaves;
Fresh watermelon cubes;

Instructions
1. In a pitcher, mix fresh mint leaves and cubes of watermelon.

2. Pour water into the pitcher.

3. For a cool, hydrating beverage, let it steep in the refrigerator.

Snack Concepts
Baked cinnamon apple slices

Ingredients

- Thinly sliced apples - Cinnamon
- Honey (if desired)

Instructions

1. Set the oven's temperature to 350°F (175°C).

2. On a baking sheet, arrange apple slices.

3. Add cinnamon and honey (if wanted) as garnishes.

4. Bake the apples for 15 to 20 minutes, or until they are soft.

5. Take pleasure in it as a warm, naturally sweet snack.

Celery with almond cream cheese

Ingredients
- Carrot sticks
- Plain and low-fat almond cream cheese

Instructions

1. Cover celery sticks with almond cream cheese.

2. Enjoy the contrast between crunchy and creamy.

Roasted chickpeas

Ingredients
chickpeas (cooked or in a can),
olive oil,
paprika, and
cumin
(to taste), salt and pepper

Instructions
1. Set the oven's temperature to 400°F (200°C).

2. Combine olive oil, paprika, cumin, salt, and pepper with the chickpeas.

3. Roast the chickpeas for 20 to 25 minutes, or until they are crispy.

4. Enjoy it as a crispy, protein-rich snack.

Dessert Selections
Banana Oat Cookies

Ingredients
ripe bananas,
mashed oats,
cinnamon, and
dark chocolate chips (optional; 70% cacao or higher)

Instructions
1. Combine mashed bananas with rolled oats, a dash of cinnamon, and any desired amount of dark chocolate chips.

2. Scoop them out into little cookies, then put them on a baking pan.

3. Bake the cookies for 15-20 minutes, or until they are firm, at 350°F (175°C).

4. Enjoy it as a dessert, free of guilt.

Mixed Berry Sorbet

Ingredients
- A variety of berries, such as strawberries, blueberries, and raspberries
Citrus juice
- Honey, if desired

Instructions
1. Blend the mixed berries with a little lemon juice and optional honey.

2. Freeze until just barely solid.

3. Use it as a delicious, delightful sorbet.

Beverages
Golden Milk with Turmeric and Ginger

Ingredients
Ground fresh ginger root;
turmeric;
unsweetened almond milk;

pepper; black;
honey, if desired

Instructions

1. In a saucepan, combine the turmeric, freshly grated ginger, almond milk, a dash of black pepper, and any optional honey.

2. Warm up, but avoid boiling.

3. Drink this anti-inflammatory and nutritious golden milk.

Strawberry and basil-infused water

Ingredients
- Sliced fresh strawberries
- Fresh basil
- Water

Instructions

1. In a pitcher, combine fresh strawberry slices and basil leaves.

2. Pour water into the pitcher.

3. Allow it to steep in the refrigerator for a tasty and fragrant beverage.

Snack concepts:
popcorn with herbs

Ingredients:
popcorn made with air.
- Dried herbs (such as thyme and oregano), optional nutritional yeast, and an olive oil mist.

Instructions
1. Pop plain popcorn with air.

2. Spray some olive oil on it.

3. Add nutritional yeast and dry herbs as desired for taste.

4. Snack on it for a salty and crunchy treat.

Sliced bell peppers with guacamole

Ingredients
Sliced bell peppers—
low-fat,
basic guacamole, either homemade or purchased

Instructions
1. Guacamole-dip bell pepper slices.

2. Enjoy the flavorful marriage of smooth guacamole and crunchy bell peppers.

Quinoa and cucumber salad

Ingredients
- Quinoa that has been cooked
- Diced cucumber
- Fresh dill
- Lemon juice
- Oil of olives
- To taste, salt and pepper

Instructions

1. Combine the cooked quinoa with the chopped cucumber, fresh dill, olive oil, lemon juice, and salt and pepper.

2. Mix everything well.

3. Snack on it for a light and revitalizing treat.

Dessert Selections:
Banana and blueberry frozen yogurt

Ingredients
ripe bananas, frozen in slices;
low-fat plain Greek yogurt; and
fresh blueberries;
honey, if desired

Instructions
1. Blend Greek yogurt, frozen banana slices, and optional honey until smooth.

2. Add fresh blueberries and fold them in.

3. If you'd like a harder texture, freeze.

4. Treat yourself to some delicious, creamy frozen yogurt.

Rice pudding with cinnamon, served chilled

Ingredients
rice pudding, either handmade or purchased, prepared with almond milk.
Cinnamon powder;
optional sliced almonds

Instructions
1. Serve rice pudding cold.

2. Add some cinnamon powder and, if wanted, chopped almonds.

3. Savor it as a cooling dessert that is comfortable.

Beverages:
Freshly squeezed orange juice

Ingredients
oranges in season.

Instructions
1. To produce natural orange juice, squeeze fresh oranges.

2. Serve chilled for a revitalizing beverage that is vitamin-rich.

Mint and Lemon Verbena Infused Water

Ingredients
- Lemon verbena leaves
- Water
- Fresh mint leaves

Instructions
1. In a pitcher, mix lemon verbena and fresh mint leaves.

2. Pour water into the pitcher.

3. Allow it to steep in the refrigerator for a flavorful and energizing beverage.

Snack Concepts:
Sliced pears with almond butter

Ingredients
- Sliced ripe pears
- Unsweetened almond butter

Instructions
1. Apply almond butter to slices of pears.

2. Enjoy the flavorful marriage of sweet pear and creamy almond butter.

Cherry tomato and mozzarella skewers

Ingredients
- Fresh mozzarella balls (bocconcini)
- Cherry tomatoes
- Fresh basil
- Optional balsamic glaze

Instructions

1. Toss fresh mozzarella balls, cherry tomatoes, and basil leaves onto skewers.

2. If desired, drizzle with a balsamic glaze.

3. Take pleasure in it as a tasty, bite-sized snack.

Roasted almonds with rosemary

Ingredients
- Olive oil
- Sea salt
- Fresh rosemary leaves
- Unsalted almonds

Instructions

1. Combine almonds with some olive oil, sea salt, and fresh rosemary leaves.

2. Roast for approximately 10 minutes at 350°F (175°C) or until aromatic.

3. After cooling, eat it as a flavorful and fragrant snack.

Dessert Selections
Berry Parfait with Yogurt

Ingredients

A combination of berries (such as blueberries and raspberries);
- Low-fat Greek yogurt;
- Honey, if desired

Instructions

1. In a glass or dish, combine low-fat Greek yogurt with mixed berries.

2. If preferred, drizzle with honey for added sweetness.

3. Enjoy it as a fruity, creamy dessert.

Chocolate Avocado Mousse

Ingredients

A mature avocado;
dark chocolate powder;
honey; and vanilla extract are optional.

Instructions
1. Combine ripe avocado, honey, unsweetened cocoa powder, and vanilla extract (if using) in a blender and process until smooth.

2. Place it in the fridge to cool.

3. Devour like an indulgent and creamy chocolate mousse.

Beverages
Iced Lemonade with Lavender

Ingredients
Lemon juice;
fresh lavender buds;
honey, if desired;
cubes of ice

Instructions

1. To create lavender tea, steep fresh lavender buds in boiling water.

2. Include honey (if preferred) and lemon juice.

3. For a fragrant and energizing lemonade, chill and serve over ice.

Pineapple and ginger-infused water

Ingredients
Fresh ginger slices
Fresh pineapple chunks
Water

Instructions
1. In a pitcher, combine fresh pineapple chunks and fresh ginger slices.

2. Pour water into the pitcher.

3. Put it in the refrigerator to steep for a refreshing beverage with a tropical flavor.

Cucumber and mint cooler

Ingredients
Slices of fresh cucumber;
fresh mint; and
sparkling water

Instructions
1. Put mint leaves and fresh cucumber slices in a glass.

2. Pour sparkling water into the glass.

3. Drink this refreshing cucumber-mint cooler to energize you.

330

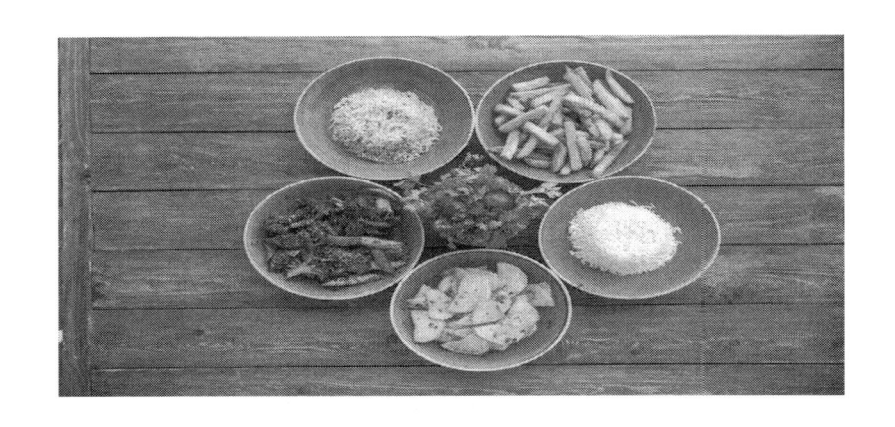

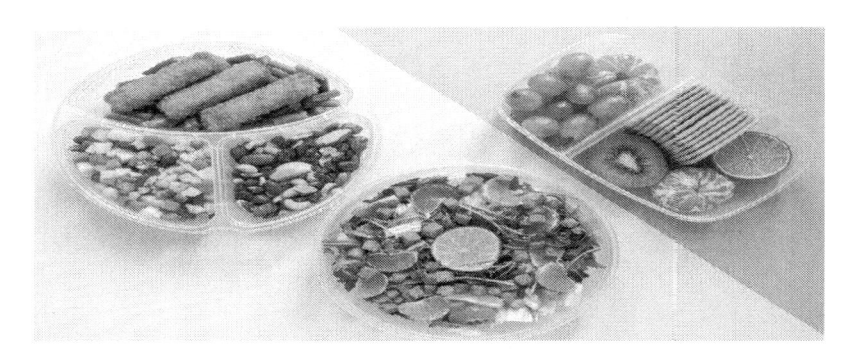

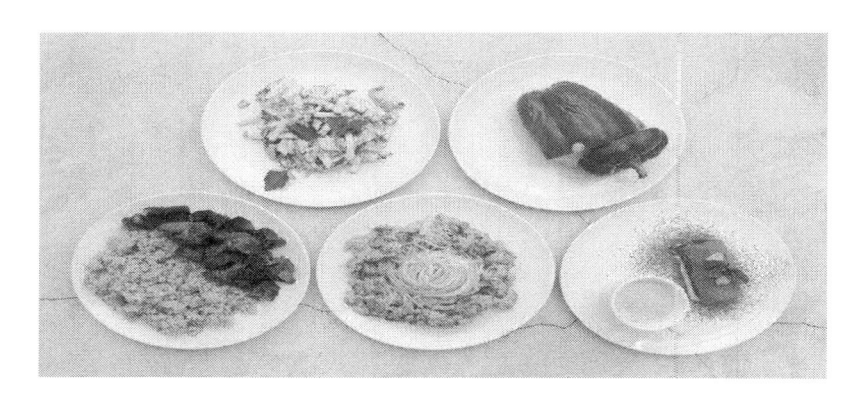

CHAPTER EIGHT

Nutritional Information and Portion Sizes

When treating gastritis or other dietary issues, understanding dietary data and serving quantities is essential. You may maintain a balanced, gastritis-friendly diet by making wise decisions. Here is a thorough breakdown of dietary data and serving sizes:

Information about nutrition: Food labels often include nutritional information, which gives important insights about a product's composition.

The following are significant elements of nutritional data:

Serving Size

1: The quantity of food on which the nutrition data are based is indicated by the serving size.

To achieve a correct nutrition evaluation, you must compare this serving size to the amount you plan to consume.

2. Calories: Calories represent the amount of energy a meal contains. Understanding calorie content may help you regulate portion sizes and keep a healthy weight in order to treat gastritis.

3. Among the macronutrients are:

Protein: vital for general health and tissue repair. Choose lean protein sources like tofu, fish, and chicken.

Carbohydrates: They provide you energy. For long-lasting energy, choose complex carbs like whole grains.

Fats are essential for good health in general. Choose healthy fats like those in avocados, almonds, and olive oil instead of unhealthy ones.

4. Fiber: Fiber helps maintain good intestinal health. Include foods high in fiber in your diet, such as fruits, vegetables, and whole grains.

5. Sugars Adding sweets in excess might aggravate gastritis symptoms. Check the ingredient list for sources of added sugars.

6. Sodium: A high-salt diet may make gastritis worse. Choose lower-sodium selections and keep an eye on salt levels, particularly in processed meals.

7. Nutritional supplements: Pay close attention to vitamins and minerals, particularly vitamin C, which some people with gastritis may find irritating.

Dimensions of portions: The quantity of food you decide to consume in one sitting is referred to as a portion size. In order to avoid overeating and lessen gastrointestinal distress, managing gastroenteritis often requires portion control.

The following is advice on portion control:

1. Use Measuring Tools: Especially for items like grains, proteins, and snacks, measuring cups and kitchen scales may help you correctly determine portion sizes.

2. Visual Cues: Acquire the skill of visual portion estimation. A 3-ounce portion of beef, for instance, is about the size of a deck of cards.

3. Plate Construction: On your plate, aim to place half of your veggies, a quarter of lean protein, and a quarter of nutritious grains or starchy vegetables.

4. Avoid supersizing: Restaurants often provide bigger quantities, so be aware of this. To share your dinner, think about splitting a dish or ordering takeout.

5. Mindful Consumption: Pay attention to the signs of hunger and fullness. Eat mindfully and quit when you are full but not stuffed.

6. To avoid mindless snacking, split food into tiny containers or bags in advance. Nuts, yogurt, or fruit are examples of healthy snack alternatives.

7. Beverages Be mindful of beverage portion amounts, particularly for sugary or caffeinated drinks. Choose modest portions, water, or herbal tea instead.

8. Listen to Your Body: Determine portion proportions in accordance with your specific requirements and hunger. Everybody doesn't need the same quantity of food.

Nutrition and Gastritis Management in Balance:

Making decisions that promote the health of your stomach while satisfying your dietary requirements is key to managing nutrition and gastritis. *Here are some useful tactics:*

1. Variation: To ensure you obtain a range of nutrients, include a variety of foods in your diet.

2. Modification: Eat things that can cause symptoms sparingly. Controlling portions may reduce pain.

3. Personalization: Modify your diet to account for any food sensitivities or triggers you may have for gastritis. To keep track of the things that make your symptoms worse, keep a food journal.

4. Consult a Dietitian: If necessary, speak with a qualified dietitian who can help you develop a customized food plan that fits your nutritional needs and aims to manage your gastritis.

5. Make Dietary Changes Gradually: Do so to allow your body time to adjust and lessen the chance of overpowering your stomach.

Understanding dietary guidelines and serving sizes gives you the ability to make decisions that support digestive health, improve your general wellbeing, and help you manage your gastritis.

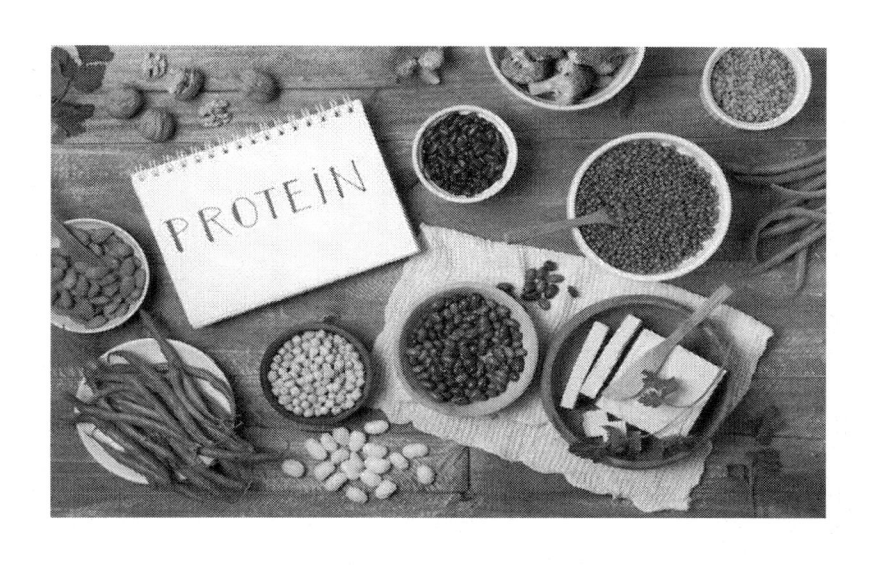

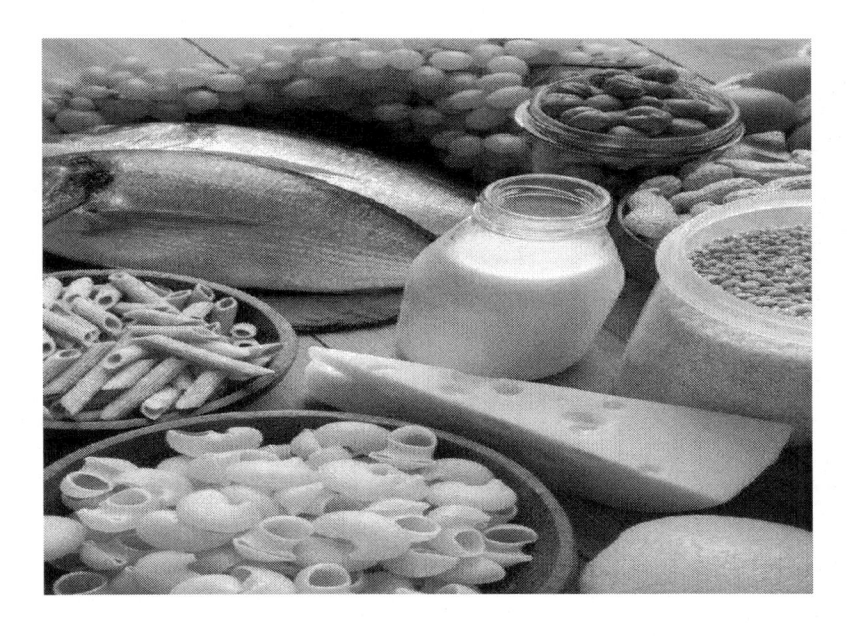

CHAPTER NINE

Tips for Dining Out with Gastritis: Gastritis-Friendly Substitutions

It might be difficult to navigate restaurant eating when you have gastritis, but you can still enjoy meals while reducing pain if you make some wise decisions and alternatives. Following are some recommendations for creating gastritis-friendly substitutes and dining out with gastritis:

1. Select the right restaurant: Give preference to eateries with a diverse menu that includes straightforward foods. - Seek out restaurants that are open to modifying dishes to meet your dietary requirements.

2. Review the menu online: Before you go, go through the menu at the restaurant's website. This enables you to select gastritis-friendly alternatives and prepare your meal in advance.

3. Select mild and straightforward dishes. To prevent irritating the lining of your stomach, choose moderate and non-spicy alternatives. - Choose foods like baked fish, grilled chicken, or steamed veggies.

4. Never be afraid to request adjustments from your server to fit your demands. For instance, ask for no hot sauces or spices.

5. Steer clear of fried and fatty meals. These foods might aggravate the symptoms of gastritis. Instead, choose foods that can be baked, grilled, or broiled.

6. Avoid Alcohol and Caffeine: Both alcohol and caffeine may make symptoms of gastritis worse. Choose non-citrus drinks, water, or herbal tea instead.

7. Take Care with Sauces and Dressings: Request sauces and dressings to be served on the side so you may regulate how much you use.

Think about replacing creamy or acidic dressings with vinegar and olive oil.

8. Opt for Gastritis-Friendly Sides: Opt for side dishes like plain rice, steamed veggies, or a straightforward salad rather than french fries or spicy coleslaw.

9. Monitoring Portion Sizes: Pay attention to portion proportions since eating too much will strain your stomach more. Think about sharing an entrée or ordering an appetizer.

10. Split desserts with others or skip them: Sugar and fat content in desserts may make gastritis symptoms worse. Think about splitting a dessert or choosing fresh fruit.

11. Engage in Mindful Eating: Take your time and enjoy every meal. Overeating may be avoided, and digestion may be aided by doing this.

12. Keep a modest snack in your luggage, such as simple crackers or a banana, in case you need something secure to eat in between meals.

13. Communicate your nutritional needs: Do not be reluctant to explain to your server your dietary limitations and the circumstances surrounding them.

14. They often provide beneficial advice. Be ready for important occasions by contacting the restaurant in advance to discuss your dietary requirements and, if required, to order a customized dish.

15. Pay Attention to Your Body: Pay attention to how your body responds to various meals and change your selections as necessary. The causes of gastritis might vary somewhat across individuals.

You may have pleasure in eating out while successfully controlling your gastritis if you use these suggestions and make intelligent adjustments. To guarantee a nice and comfortable eating experience for people with gastritis, keep in mind that contact with restaurant employees is essential. Don't be hesitant to speak about your dietary requirements either.

Tips for Eating Out While Having Gastroenteritis

While eating out with gastritis might be difficult, you can still enjoy restaurant meals while avoiding pain if you make some wise decisions and exercise attentiveness. Here are some helpful pointers:

1. "Plan Ahead" by doing some internet research on the restaurant's menu before you attend. Look for foods that may be altered to suit your requirements or ones that are suitable for people with gastritis.

2. Select mild dishes: Choose meals that are light, uncomplicated, and not very seasoned or

spicy. Proteins like chicken or fish that are grilled or baked are often good selections.

3. Pose inquiries. Never be afraid to ask your waiter about the ingredients and techniques used to prepare a meal. Make adjustments, such as asking for grilled rather than fried food or requesting to avoid hot sauces.

4. 'Portion Control' Restaurant portions are often enormous. To prevent overeating, think about splitting a meal with a dining buddy or requesting a half-sized quantity.

5. Steer clear of trigger foods. Avoid foods that are known to be triggers, such as citrus, tomatoes, onions, and spicy meals. Be careful while using sauces and condiments since they might contain unidentified allergens.

6. Avoid carbonated beverages: Drinks with carbonation may make your stomach feel worse. Instead, choose herbal tea, still water, or non-citrus fruit juices.

7. Mindful Eating: Take your time and enjoy every meal. This not only helps with digestion but also with fullness recognition, limiting overeating.

8. Considerations for salad: Salads may be a healthy option, but use caution when using acidic dressings. Use the dressing sparingly and ask for it on the side. Avoid eating raw onion and tomato salads.

9. Roasted or Steamed Vegetables: Steamed or roasted veggies are good side dishes to choose from since they are often easier on the stomach than fried or spicy ones.

10. Grain-based dishes and starchy sides Choose simple pasta, rice, or baked potatoes without additional toppings. These might provide a tasty foundation for your dinner.

11. Alternatives to dessert Dessert alternatives like fresh fruit, sorbet, or plain yogurt may be

less grating than rich, creamy desserts or citrus-based treats.

12. "Take Your Time": Don't eat quickly. While your stomach is processing the meal, enjoy the company and conversation.

13. Moderation with alcohol If you decide to drink alcohol, do so sparingly. Instead of cocktails with citrus or fizzy mixers, wine or mild beer may be easier to handle.

14. Bring Digestive Aids: In case of sudden pain, think about carrying digestive aids like antacids or prescription drugs.

15. Be Prepared: Despite your best efforts, unforeseen irritants may still make an appearance in your meal. Have relief on hand and be ready for any unexpected pain. You may enjoy eating out with gastritis without losing your pleasure or well-being if you use these suggestions and make wise decisions.

Keep in mind that everyone has different triggers and tolerances, so it's important to pay attention to your body and choose things that suit you the best. You may control symptoms and improve stomach health by incorporating food changes that are favorable to those with gastritis. Here are a few such replacements to think about:

1. Replace refined grains with whole grains instead of white bread, rice, and pasta to enhance fiber content and improve digestion.

2. Lean Proteins for Fatty Meats: To lower the risk of irritation, choose lean cuts of meat, poultry, and fish instead of fatty cuts.

3. Plant-Based Milk for Dairy: If dairy causes pain, consider lactose-free or plant-based milk alternatives like almond, soy, or oat milk.

4. Herbs for Spices: Instead of using hot spices that might upset the stomach, season food with herbs like basil, oregano, and rosemary.

5. Use olive oil instead of butter when cooking and topping foods to lower your consumption of saturated fats.

6. Fresh Fruit for Citrus: Substitute non-acidic fruits like bananas, melons, and apples for citrus fruits like oranges and grapefruits.

7. Non-Citrus Juices: Opt for fruit juices other than citrus, such as apple, pear, or berry juices, rather than acidic drinks like orange or grapefruit juice.

8. Use moderate condiments instead of spiciness or acidity, such as honey, mustard, or dressings made with yogurt.

9. Choose low-fat or fat-free dairy products instead of full-fat dairy to lower the amount of fat that may cause gastritis symptoms.

10. Cooked veggies, as opposed to raw ones, are simpler to digest than raw vegetables like broccoli, carrots, and spinach.

11. Water for Carbonated Drinks: To reduce extra gas and irritation, drink still water instead of carbonated drinks.

12. Ginger Tea for Caffeine: Opt for caffeine-free herbal teas or ginger tea instead of irritable coffee or black tea.

13. Choose plain, unsweetened yogurt and flavor it with your preferred fruit instead of flavored yogurt that has already been sweetened.

14. "Bland Snacks": Choose bland snacks instead of spicy or highly seasoned ones, such as rice cakes, plain crackers, or unsalted pretzels.

15. Almond or sunflower seed butter: almond or sunflower seed butter may be used in place of peanut butter, which some people may find more difficult to digest.

16. Baking soda for antacids: Use baking soda diluted in water as a natural antacid if advised to

do so by your doctor. Individual tolerances might differ; therefore, it's important to be aware of how your body responds to various alternatives.

You can find the best replacements for treating your gastritis symptoms by keeping a meal diary. Personalized advice on making the right dietary modifications may also be obtained by speaking with a healthcare professional or nutritionist.

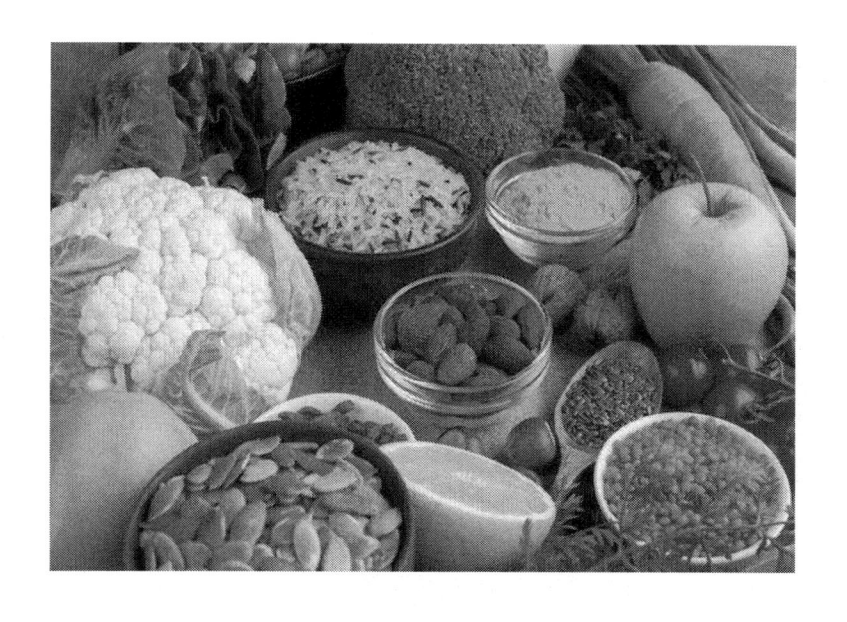

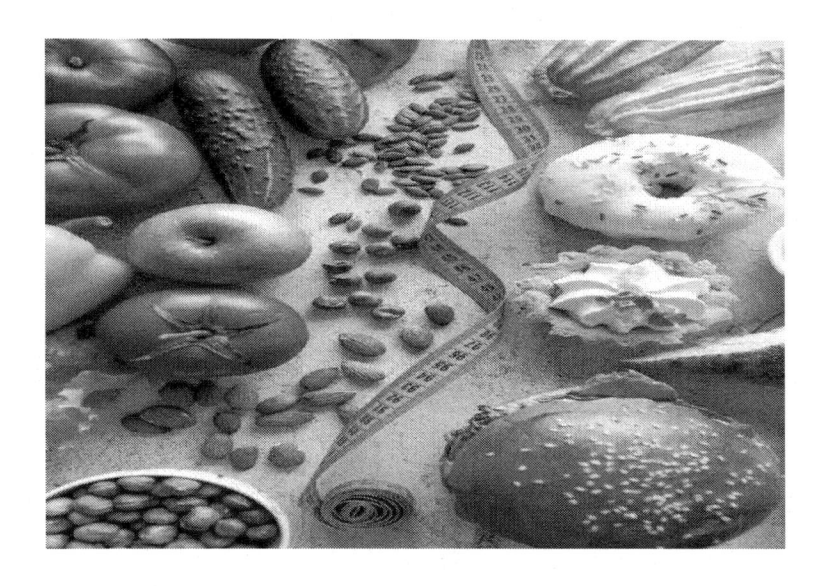

CHAPTER TEN

Gastritis Management and Lifestyle

Your quality of life may be greatly enhanced by controlling your gastritis and making the required lifestyle adjustments. Here are some essential tactics and advice for managing gastritis effectively:

1. Dietary Modifications: Adhere to a low-acid, non-spicy diet that is suitable for those with gastritis. Steer clear of trigger foods, including fried, spicy, acidic, and highly processed meals. Eat smaller meals more often to lessen gastrointestinal discomfort. Include fiber-rich meals to improve stomach health and assist with digestion.

2. Hydration: Drink plenty of water to be properly hydrated and to calm the stomach lining. Limit your intake of alcohol and coffee since they might irritate your stomach.

3. Stress Reduction: Use relaxation methods like deep breathing, meditation, or yoga to manage stress. Finding methods to relax is essential since gastritis symptoms may be made worse by high levels of stress.

4. Medication: Take drugs, such as proton pump inhibitors (PPIs) or antacids, as instructed if given by a medical expert. Attend follow-up visits and adhere to the prescribed course of therapy.

5. Smoking Cessation: If you smoke, giving it up may greatly improve the symptoms of gastritis and your general health.

6. Alcohol should only be used in moderation since it might irritate the stomach lining.

7. Avoiding NSAIDs since they may make gastritis worse. Examples of NSAIDs are ibuprofen and aspirin. If you need other pain treatment methods, speak to a doctor.

8. Consistent Exercise: Exercise often to maintain a healthy weight and advance general wellbeing.

9. Identifying Triggers: Keep a food journal to note which meals or drinks make your symptoms worse. - Avoiding these triggers will reduce pain.

10. Adequate Sleep: Make sure you receive enough restful sleep, since it's important for recovery and general wellness.

11. Stay informed on the origins, symptoms, and possible complications of gastritis. Keep up-to-date with the suggestions and counsel given by your healthcare practitioner.

12. Schedule regular check-ups with your healthcare practitioner to monitor your condition and, if required, modify your treatment plan. Consult a certified dietitian.

13. Consider seeking the advice of a certified dietitian who can assist you in developing a custom gastritis diet plan.

14. Gradual dietary adjustments: Give your body time to adapt by making dietary changes gradually. Practice mindful eating by paying attention to how you chew your food and how much you enjoy each mouthful.

15. Social Support: Consider joining a support group for people with digestive disorders or asking friends and family for help.

Keep in mind that managing gastritis may require persistence and patience. Working together with your healthcare physician can help you create a personalized strategy that will meet your unique requirements and guarantee the greatest results.

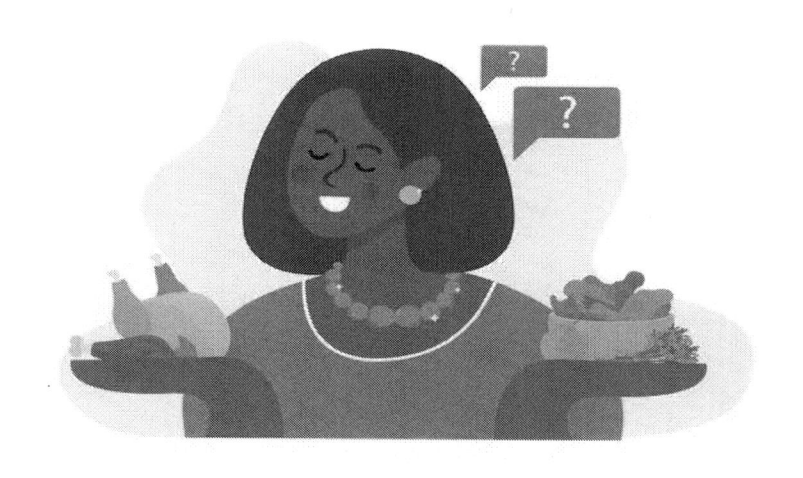

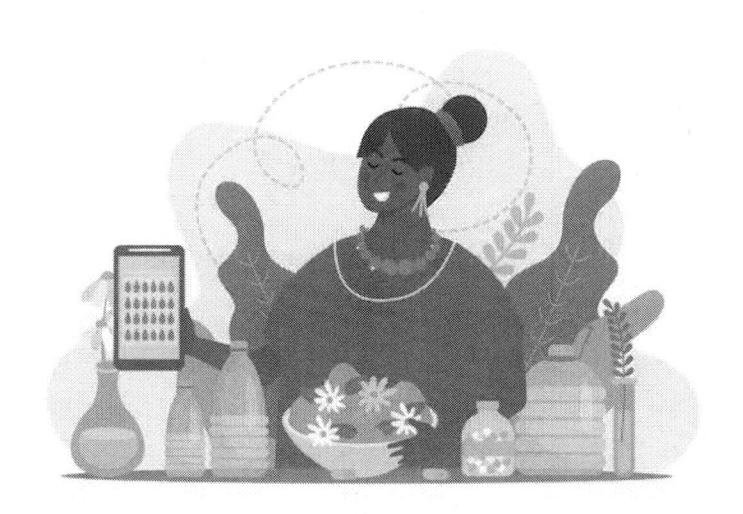

CHAPTER ELEVEN

Frequently Asked Questions and Answers

1. Gastritis: What is it?

Gastritis is an inflammation of the stomach's lining that may cause pain and discomfort during digestion.

2. Why does gastritis occur?

A number of things, including drinking too much alcohol, using NSAIDs for an extended period of time, stress, and bacterial infections (such as H. pylori), may lead to gastritis.

3. Can diet aid in gastritis management?

Yes, by lowering inflammation and eliminating items that aggravate symptoms, a well-planned diet may aid in managing gastritis.

4. What typical gastritis symptoms are there?

Abdominal discomfort, bloating, nausea, vomiting, and a burning feeling in the stomach are all typical symptoms of gastritis.

5. Is there a special diet to follow for gastritis?

There is no one-size-fits-all gastritis diet, but there are basic rules to go by, such as staying away from alcohol, spicy meals, and foods high in acid.

6. With gastritis, what foods should I avoid?

Spicy meals, citrus fruits, tomatoes, caffeine, alcohol, fried and fatty foods, and carbonated drinks are among the foods to stay away from.

7. What meals are good for people with gastritis?

Lean proteins, whole grains, non-citrus fruits, vegetables, ginger, and meals high in fiber are among the foods that are good for those with gastroenteritis.

8. Is it okay to eat dairy products if you have gastritis?

While it's possible to eat dairy products in moderation, it's recommended to go for low-fat or nonfat varieties and pay attention to how your body responds.

9. Can someone with gastritis drink coffee or tea?

Coffee and caffeinated teas should be used in moderation or avoided as they might cause gastrointestinal irritation and increase the production of stomach acid.

10. Are there certain spices and herbs that may treat gastritis?

Yes, the anti-inflammatory qualities of chamomile, ginger, and turmeric make them effective remedies for gastritis.

11. Can someone with gastritis consume alcohol?

Alcohol should be avoided or used very sparingly since it might increase the symptoms of gastritis and harm the lining of the stomach.

12. How can I treat my gastritis when eating out?

Pick simple meals while eating out, ask for no hot ingredients, and request dressings and sauces on the side.

13. What culinary techniques are suited to people with gastritis?

For gastritis-friendly foods, baking, grilling, steaming, and sautéing with little to no oil are ideal cooking techniques.

14. With gastritis, is it important to eat smaller, more frequent meals?

Eating smaller, more frequent meals might help you control the symptoms of gastritis and avoid overfilling your stomach.

15. Does stress make the symptoms of gastritis worse?

Yes, stress may worsen the symptoms of gastritis; thus, practicing stress reduction strategies like deep breathing and meditation might be helpful.

16. How long does it take for dietary adjustments to cure gastritis?

The recovery from gastritis may take anywhere from a few weeks to a few months, although dietary adjustments can help within that time frame.

17. With gastritis, should I abstain from all acidic foods?

Even though it's ideal to restrict acidic meals, not all acidic foods have the same effects on different people, so you may need to pinpoint your own triggers.

18. Can someone with gastritis drink dairy substitutes like almond milk?

Almond milk, for example, may be a fine dairy substitute; just make sure they are unflavored and unsweetened.

19. Are sparkling drinks and carbonated water healthy for those who have gastritis?

It's advisable to consume carbonated drinks in moderation or to stay away from them altogether since they might cause bloating and discomfort.

20. Can someone with gastritis eat chocolate?

Chocolate should only be taken in moderation since it contains a lot of fat and caffeine, both of which may irritate the lining of the stomach.

21. How can someone with gastritis remain hydrated?

You may keep hydrated without exacerbating gastritis by consuming water, herbal teas, and non-citrus, non-caffeinated drinks.

22. Can I consume spicy cuisine if H. Is Pylori the cause of my gastritis? infected with pylori?

Even if H is the source of your gastritis, you should avoid spicy meals. pylori because they might make the inflammation worse.

23. Are over-the-counter antacids safe to use for gastritis? Over-the-counter antacids may provide short-term comfort, but a doctor should be consulted for a thorough diagnosis and treatment strategy.

24. What should I do if I unintentionally eat a meal that causes gastritis?

If you accidentally eat a trigger meal, pay attention to how your body responds and think about maintaining a food journal to track your triggers.

25. Can gastritis cause more serious digestive problems?

Gastritis must be managed with dietary changes and medical guidance since it may worsen if left untreated.

26. Are there certain foods that might aid in gastritis prevention?

A well-balanced diet full of fresh produce, whole grains, lean proteins, and other nutrients may improve digestive health and lower the risk of gastritis.

27. How can I stop my gastritis from getting worse?

Maintaining a gastritis-friendly diet, controlling stress, and avoiding identified triggers are necessary for preventing flare-ups.

28. Can gastritis be treated just with diet?

Dietary adjustments may help manage some instances of gastritis and lessen symptoms, but treating the underlying cause may be necessary for a full recovery.

29. For advice on a gastritis diet, should I speak with a nutritionist?

Speaking with a nutritionist or dietitian might be helpful since they can provide specialized nutritional advice based on your unique requirements.

30. Can dietary supplements for herbs treat gastritis?

Although certain herbal supplements, such as slippery elm and licorice root, are thought to have calming benefits for the stomach, speak with a doctor before taking any herbal products.

31. Is maintaining a gastritis diet vital even after symptoms subside?

Maintaining symptom alleviation and advancing long-term stomach health may both be achieved by sticking to a gastritis-friendly diet.

32. Are there any dietary suggestions in particular for kids with gastritis? Diets for kids with gastritis should consist of light, simple meals that are easy to digest.

33. Does gastritis influence the absorption of nutrients?

Yes, gastritis may affect how well nutrients are absorbed, so it's crucial to prioritize nutrient-rich diets and, if required, supplements.

34. Is it okay to eat yogurt and other fermented foods while having gastritis?

Consuming plain, non-fat yogurt containing live bacteria in moderation may be beneficial for gut health.

35. Can dietary allergies or sensitivities cause gastritis?

Food allergies or sensitivities may exacerbate the symptoms of gastritis; therefore, it's critical to recognize and stay away from trigger foods.

36. How can I avoid getting gastritis while I'm out to eat or traveling?

Research gastritis-friendly choices in your location and make specific requests at eateries before you go or eat out.

37. Can someone with gastritis drink alcohol-free beer or wine?

For some people, alcohol-free beer or wine may be a safer alternative, but it's important to verify the components for any possible triggers.

38. Does using probiotic pills help treat gastritis?

Probiotic pills may help balance intestinal flora, but before taking them, talk to a doctor since everyone's body reacts differently.

39. Can gastritis run in families?

Since gastritis may have a hereditary component, it's a good idea to talk to your doctor about any family members who have had stomach problems.

40. Is there a relationship between GERD and gastritis?

The symptoms of both gastroesophageal reflux disease (GERD) and acid reflux sometimes overlap, and persistent gastritis may enhance this risk.

41. How can I make these recipes for gastritis vegetarian or vegan-friendly?

A lot of the recipes in this cookbook may be modified by using plant-based proteins instead, such as tofu, tempeh, or legumes.

42. If I have strong tastes, may I add herbs and spices to these recipes?

You may experiment with adding herbs and spices to these dishes to improve the taste, but start off slowly and stay away from too-spicy alternatives.

43. Are there any particular dishes that are good for kids with gastritis?

This cookbook has several milder recipes that may be appropriate for kids with gastritis, such as basic pasta with a light sauce or straightforward rice meals.

44. Can someone with gastritis eat dessert?

Desserts should only be eaten in moderation, and you should try to choose ones that are created with gastritis-friendly components, such as fruit-based desserts or yogurt parfaits.

45. Can I utilize these recipes to save time throughout the week by meal-prepping?

Yes, many of these foods may be prepared in advance, making it simpler to follow your gastritis-friendly diet throughout the hectic workweek.

46. Is a gastroenterologist important for the treatment of gastritis?

A gastroenterologist can help determine the underlying cause of your chronic or severe gastritis symptoms and help you create a treatment plan.

47. Can someone with gastritis drink herbal teas like chamomile or peppermint?

Lower esophageal sphincter relaxation from peppermint tea may make symptoms worse. In general, chamomile tea is softer and can be a better option. Daily management of gastritis.

48 How can I manage the signs of gastritis when pregnant?

Consulting a healthcare professional for safe medication choices and pregnancy-appropriate dietary changes may be necessary to manage gastritis during pregnancy.

49 Can gastritis affect the quality of my sleep?

Gastritis symptoms, such as pain at night, might impair sleep. It could be beneficial to elevate your upper body as you sleep or have a little snack before bed.

50. Is it okay to consume uncooked produce while you have gastritis?

Although eating fresh fruits and vegetables is typically healthy, some people with gastritis may find it difficult to digest them. To make them more gastrointestinal-friendly, softly steam them or cook them.

51. Can practices for reducing stress, such as yoga or meditation, assist with gastritis?

By easing stress-related symptoms, stress management approaches may support the treatment of gastritis. It could be advantageous to include relaxing techniques into your daily routine.

52. What are some doable strategies for maintaining a diet that is gastritis-friendly when traveling?

When traveling, bring gastritis-friendly foods, look out for acceptable eateries in your destination city, and, if necessary, take digestive aids.

53. Can gastritis harm the condition of my teeth?

Dental problems, including enamel degradation, might result from gastritis-related frequent vomiting. After vomiting, rinsing your mouth with water may help safeguard your teeth.

54. Is it necessary to abstain from all alcoholic beverages, including wine and beer?

Although it's best to keep alcohol intake to a minimum, some people could do better with a little wine or beer than strong liquor. Keep an eye on your body's response.

55. Can mood swings and irritation be brought on by gastritis?

Chronic gastritis may cause mood swings since it makes everyday living uncomfortable and difficult. Symptom management may enhance general wellbeing.

56. If neglected, might gastritis result in complications?

It is crucial to address and manage gastritis since it has the potential to cause problems like stomach ulcers or bleeding.

57. Is it okay to provide probiotics to kids who have gastritis?

Before giving probiotics to kids with gastritis, talk to a doctor since the right strain and dose depend on the child's age and health.

58. Can gastritis make someone eat-averse?

Discomfort brought on by gastroenteritis may trigger momentary dietary aversions.

Reintroducing tolerable foods gradually might aid in overcoming these dislikes.

59. How can I help a family member who has gastritis?

Show compassion and understanding, assist with food preparation, and motivate them to heed medical recommendations and have a gastritis-friendly lifestyle.

60. Can elderly people with gastritis still absorb nutrients?

The necessity of a nutrient-rich diet is highlighted by the possibility that older people have a greater risk of nutrient malabsorption owing to gastritis.

61. Can irritable bowel syndrome (IBS) or other digestive problems like gastritis be connected to each other?

Since both gastroenteritis and IBS entail digestive symptoms, they may coexist. A healthcare provider's accurate diagnosis and treatment may distinguish between the two.

62. Is it possible to take certain foods that are good for gastritis too much and have symptoms get worse?

Even meals that are good for people with gastritis should not be consumed in excess. The key is moderation and controlling portions.

63. Can gastritis damage my body's future tolerance to spicy foods?

Even when symptoms subside, chronic gastritis may leave your stomach more susceptible to spicy meals, so it's best to proceed cautiously.

64. How can someone with gastritis negotiate social events and gatherings?

Inform hosts of your food requirements and choose gastritis-friendly choices while attending events. Place more emphasis on mingling than just eating.

65. Can gastritis interfere with my capacity to continue exercising?

While acute symptoms may momentarily restrict physical activity, eating a gastritis-friendly diet may boost your general level of energy and exercise program.

66. Can chronic gastritis result in nutritional deficiencies?

Long-term gastritis may result in nutritional deficits. You may avoid this by regularly evaluating your diet and making dietary changes.

67. How can I treat the symptoms of gastritis when I'm menstruating?

Menstrual hormone fluctuations might make gastritis symptoms worse. Keeping hydrated especially with warm water and selecting soft meals may ease pain.

68. Is it desirable to have an endoscopy or other test for gastritis on a frequent basis?

Your healthcare practitioner should decide the frequency of diagnostic tests like endoscopy depending on your unique condition and requirements.

69. Can thyroid issues or other chronic illnesses like diabetes be linked to gastritis?

Other medical disorders have been associated with gastritis. With your healthcare professional, go through your medical history and any possible correlations.

70. Can gastroenteritis alter bowel habits?

Gastritis mostly affects the stomach lining, although more serious instances may cause problems with digestion. If your bowel habits change, talk to your doctor.

71. How can I modify these meals for a person who has dietary intolerances or allergies?

By changing ingredients or staying away from known allergens, many of these recipes may be modified to suit allergies or intolerances.

72. Does halitosis or poor breath result from gastritis?

Gastritis may aggravate problems like acid reflux, which may contribute to foul breath. Keeping up decent dental hygiene may lessen this.

73. Can people with gastritis safely eat dairy-free ice cream?

For some people with gastritis, dairy-free ice cream may be a good treat, but be sure to check the ingredients for any possible irritants.

74. How can I manage the symptoms of gastritis when there is a lot of stress present, such as a test or a job deadline?

Give stress-reduction practices like deep breathing, meditation, and time management first priority to lessen the symptoms of gastritis caused by stress.

75. Can gastritis result in poor energy and fatigue?

Fatigue may result from chronic gastritis. Making sure you have enough food and sleep might help you fight the condition's related weariness.

76. Is it safe to attempt alternative treatments for gastritis, such as acupuncture or acupressure?

Alternative treatments could be helpful for some people, but you should always talk to a doctor before starting one.

77. Can food intolerances like lactose intolerance cause gastritis?

It's important to recognize and treat both conditions because gastroenteritis can make food intolerances worse.

78. Can gastritis interfere with my body's ability to absorb vitamins or medications?

For advice, speak with your healthcare provider if you have chronic gastritis, as it may affect how well you absorb some supplements or medications.

79. How can I deal with the frequent heartburn that comes with gastritis?

Medications prescribed by a doctor or over-the-counter antacids can help treat heartburn brought on by gastritis.

80. Is it okay for people with gastritis to eat fermented foods like kimchi or sauerkraut?

Although some people with gastritis may not be able to tolerate fermented foods, they can still have probiotic benefits. Start out slowly and pay attention to how your body reacts.

81. Can running or weightlifting make you uncomfortable when you have gastritis?

Excessive exercise, particularly after eating, might make gastritis symptoms worse. To avoid pain, schedule your workouts around mealtimes.

82. How should I treat my gastritis over the seasons and on special days?

Preparing your own food, letting hosts know about any dietary restrictions, and bringing gastritis-friendly foods are all possible ways to enjoy holiday celebrations while managing gastritis.

83. Can gastritis interfere with the body's ability to absorb vitamins and minerals from foods like fruits and vegetables?

Because inflammation associated with gastroenteritis may interfere with nutritional absorption, it's important to concentrate on a balanced diet high in fruits and vegetables.

84. Are there certain herbs or drinks that might reduce the inflammation brought on by gastritis?

Licorice root and drinks with ginger or marshmallow root may help reduce inflammation brought on by gastritis, but you should talk to your doctor first.

85. Can gastritis influence my ability to taste and appreciate food?

Gastritis may temporarily impair your perception of taste, but adopting a gastritis-friendly diet will help you continue to enjoy meals.

86. How can I control gastritis during lengthy flights or travel?

During lengthy flights or travel, remain hydrated, bring snacks, and pick gastritis-friendly alternatives while eating at airports or during layovers.

87. Can gastritis damage my mental health and well-being?

Chronic gastritis may damage mental health owing to pain and dietary limitations. Seek help from healthcare providers and mental health specialists as required.

88. Is it important to avoid all types of caffeine, even decaffeinated coffee?

While decaffeinated coffee contains less caffeine, it may still irritate the stomach lining; therefore, some people with gastritis choose to avoid it.

89. Can gastritis create symptoms like chest discomfort or trouble breathing?

Gastritis-related discomfort may sometimes be misinterpreted for chest pain or shortness of breath. For an accurate assessment, see a healthcare professional.

90. How can I modify these dishes for a person who has celiac illness or gluten sensitivity?

Many of the recipes in this cookbook may be modified for those who are gluten-intolerant by substituting gluten-free products like rice flour or oats that have received the necessary certification.

91. Can gastritis affect my appetite and sense of smell?

Your sense of smell and appetite may be briefly affected by gastroenteritis. Trying new tastes and smells might help you get your appetite back.

92. How can I control my gastritis while going to social gatherings that include a variety of cuisines?

At various social gatherings, look around and choose gastritis-friendly foods that suit your dietary requirements. Ask hosts about ingredients at any time.

93. Can my sleep patterns and sleep quality be affected by gastritis?

Heartburn or other signs of discomfort caused by gastroenteritis might interfere with sleep. Avoiding heavy meals just before bed and elevating your head as you sleep may also be beneficial.

94. Is it okay to eat food made with yogurt if you have gastritis?

Some people with gastritis may find comfort in meals made with plain yogurt; however, dishes with additional sweeteners or artificial tastes should be avoided.

95. How can I treat my gastritis while exercising or doing sports?

Maintaining hydration and eating a modest, easily digested meal before exercise may help control gastritis when engaging in physical activity.

96. Can gastritis make it harder for me to take hot spices like black pepper?

Gastritis may lower one's tolerance for hot spices. Try using softer herbs and spices to enhance tastes without causing sensitivity.

97. Can environmental factors like air pollution or allergies cause gastritis?

Although the stomach lining is the primary site of gastritis, environmental factors may affect general health. Exposure to contaminants should be minimized.

98. Can hiccups or burping be caused by gastritis?

Especially after meals, gastroenteritis may cause hiccups or frequent burping. These symptoms may be lessened by figuring out the causes and changing meal portions.

99. Puddings made with rice or almond milk are safe to eat if you have gastritis?

Puddings made with rice or almond milk may be easy on the stomach and suitable for some people who have gastritis. Pick products with a few added sugars.

100. Can gastritis harm my teeth and lead to cavities?

Cavities in the teeth can develop as a result of frequent vomiting brought on by gastritis. To avoid this, practicing good oral hygiene is crucial.

101. How can I continue eating healthfully despite food cravings or emotional eating?

Recognize the factors that lead to emotional eating and look into healthier options to satiate cravings, including a modest portion of fresh fruit or dark chocolate.

102. Can rheumatoid arthritis or other autoimmune diseases cause gastritis?

Some autoimmune diseases and gastritis may coexist. With your healthcare professional, go through your medical history and any possible correlations.

103. Can gastritis cause bloating or excessive gas?

Gastritis may make some people feel like they have too much gas. These symptoms may be lessened by controlling portion amounts and staying away from foods that cause gas.

104. How can I keep up a gastritis-friendly diet on a tight budget or with little money?

Purchasing in bulk, selecting seasonal food, and picking store brands whenever feasible are all economical gastritis-friendly choices.

105. Can gastritis alter the consistency or color of stools?

While severe instances of gastritis may cause changes in stools' color or consistency, the condition predominantly affects the stomach. If you observe these changes, speak with a healthcare professional.

106. How can I control gastritis during pregnancy without medications?

Making dietary changes, eating smaller, more frequent meals, and avoiding recognized triggers may all be necessary for treating gastritis without medication during pregnancy.

107. Can children get gastritis?

If so, how is it treated in pediatric cases? Children may get gastroenteritis, and management strategies often entail dietary adjustments, identifying triggers, and contacting a physician for the best course of action.

108. How can I treat the signs of pregnancy-related gastritis?

Consulting a healthcare professional for safe medication choices and pregnancy-appropriate dietary changes may be necessary to manage gastritis during pregnancy.

109. Can gastritis affect the quality of my sleep?

Gastritis symptoms, such as pain at night, might impair sleep. It could be beneficial to elevate your upper body as you sleep or have a little snack before bed.

110. Is it okay to consume uncooked produce while you have gastritis?

Although eating fresh fruits and vegetables is typically healthy, some people with gastritis may find it difficult to digest them. To make them more gastrointestinal-friendly, softly steam them or cook them.

111. Can practices for reducing stress, such as yoga or meditation, assist with gastritis?

By easing stress-related symptoms, stress management approaches may support the treatment of gastritis. It could be advantageous to include relaxing techniques into your daily routine.

112. What are some doable strategies for maintaining a diet that is gastritis-friendly when traveling?

When traveling, bring gastritis-friendly foods, look out for acceptable eateries in your destination city, and, if necessary, take digestive aids.

113. Can gastritis harm the condition of my teeth?

Dental problems, including enamel degradation, might result from gastritis-related frequent vomiting. After vomiting, rinsing your mouth with water may help safeguard your teeth.

114. Is it necessary to abstain from all alcoholic beverages, including wine and beer?

Although it's best to keep alcohol intake to a minimum, some people could do better with a little wine or beer than strong liquor. Keep an eye on your body's response.

115. Can mood swings and irritation be brought on by gastritis?

Chronic gastritis may cause mood swings since it makes everyday living uncomfortable and difficult. Symptom management may enhance general wellbeing.

116. If neglected, might gastritis result in complications?

It is crucial to address and manage gastritis since it has the potential to cause problems like stomach ulcers or bleeding.

117. How many probiotics can be used to treat pediatric gastritis?

Before giving probiotics to kids with gastritis, talk to a doctor since the right strain and dose depend on the child's age and health.

118. Can gastritis make someone eat-averse?

Discomfort brought on by gastroenteritis may trigger momentary dietary aversions. Reintroducing tolerable foods gradually might aid in overcoming these dislikes.

119. How can I help a family member who has gastritis?

Show compassion and understanding, assist with food preparation, and motivate them to heed medical recommendations and have a gastritis-friendly lifestyle.

120. Can elderly people with gastritis still absorb nutrients?

The necessity of a nutrient-rich diet is highlighted by the possibility that older persons have a greater risk of nutrient malabsorption owing to gastritis.

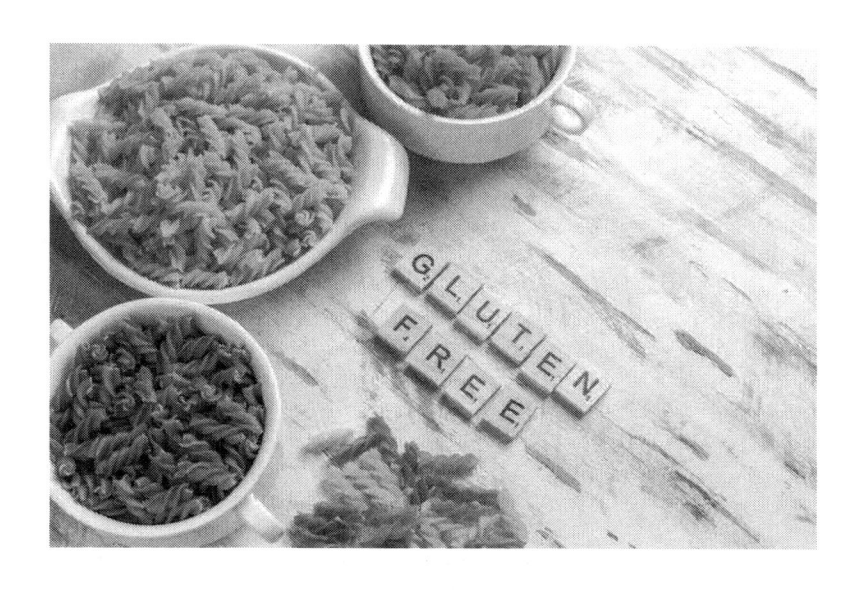

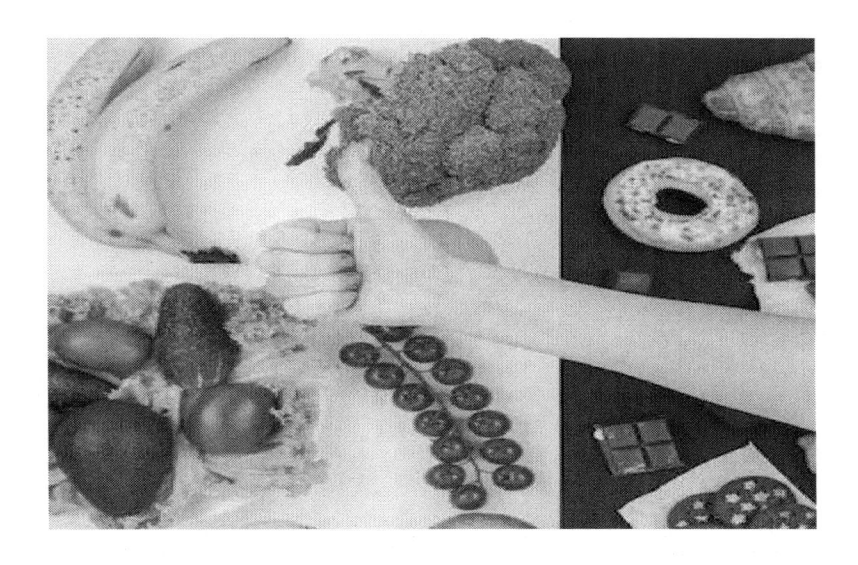

EPILOGUE

Finally, we hope that as you've journeyed through the pages of this cookbook, you've gained a restored feeling of control over your gastritis and digestive health, in addition to some delectable meals. These meals were carefully and thoughtfully created for folks who want both sustenance and respite from the pain that gastritis may cause.

You now realize that eating should be approached carefully and mindfully if you have gastropathy. It's important to consider how you eat as well as what you consume. You now have access to a variety of dishes that follow the guidelines of a gastritis-friendly diet: they are easy on the stomach, low in acidity, anti-inflammatory, and full of comforting ingredients.

You've probably noticed a repeating theme as you've read through this cookbook's chapters:

the significance of selecting foods and meals that put your stomach's health first without sacrificing taste. You've learned that eating healthily while managing your gastritis doesn't need to compromise flavor. It's about striking the proper balance, discovering new tastes, and treating your body gently.

You've come across recipes along the way that include healthy grains, lean meats, fiber-rich foods, and anti-inflammatory components. You now understand the value of including probiotics in your diet to promote gut health, as well as the therapeutic properties of herbs, spices, and other culinary ingredients. You've been given advice on maintaining your gastritis-friendly lifestyle, including how to prepare meals, go out, and make mindful adjustments.

This cookbook serves as a reminder that caring for your health is a personal and inspiring journey, in addition to providing recipes and nutritional guidance. It involves paying attention to your body, comprehending its cues, and making decisions that support wellbeing. It's about enjoying yourself in the kitchen, experimenting with tastes, and feeding loved ones healthy meals.

We advise you to keep looking into meals and cooking methods that are good for people with gastritis as time goes on. Be inventive and exploratory, and don't be afraid to change these recipes to suit your own preferences. Keep in mind that healing is a process, and over time, what works best for you can change.

We would like to close by sending you our sincere best wishes for good health and happiness. May the dishes in this cookbook not only alleviate the symptoms of gastritis but also brighten your eating experience. Accept the healing and consoling power of food, and may your path through gastritis be full of delectable discoveries and a revitalized feeling of well-being.

We appreciate you sharing with us a little of your gastritis experience. We hope your future is filled with delicious meals that are also gastritis-friendly.

Made in the USA
Columbia, SC
02 March 2025